Transform Your Skin by Identifying Your Trigger Foods and How They Affect Your Gut Microbiome, Immune System, and Hormones

THE CLEAR SKIN DIET

Unlocking the Secret Link Between Food Sensitivities and Skin Health

Maria Azizian, MD

Copyright © 2024 by Maria Azizian

All rights reserved.

ISBN: 979-8-9913755-0-4

All rights reserved. No part of this publication may be reproduced, distributed, or transmitted in any form or by any means, including photocopying, recording, or other electronic or mechanical methods, without the prior written permission of the publisher, except in the case of brief quotations embodied in critical reviews and certain other non-commercial uses permitted by copyright law.

First Edition

Library of Congress Control Number: 2024918902

Cover design idea by Rima Petrosyan

Editing supervision by Zorianna Petrosyan

Printed in the United States of America

DEDICATION

To my husband, Erin. Your unwavering support has made this journey possible.

TABLE OF CONTENTS

INTRODUCTION 1

PART I: Food Sensitivities and Skin Health 9

CHAPTER 1: Understanding Food Sensitivities:
How They Differ from Food Allergies 11

    Food Sensitivities vs. Food Allergies: The Overview 12
    Food Sensitivities vs. Food Allergies: Immunology 13
    Food Sensitivities vs. Food Allergies: Onset 14
    Food Sensitivities vs. Food Allergies: Diagnosis 15
    Food Sensitivities vs. Food Allergies: Longevity 20
    Food Sensitivities vs. Food Allergies: Half-Life 22
    Food Sensitivities vs. Food Allergies: Food Amounts Needed to Elicit a Reaction 23

CHAPTER 2: Definitions of Skin Conditions Linked to Food Sensitivities 25

    Acne 25
    Eczema 27
    Seborrheic Dermatitis 29
    Contact Dermatitis 29
    Psoriasis 30
    Rosacea 32
    Hives 34
    Types of Hives 35
    Rashes 36
    Pruritus (Itching Without a Rash) 37

PART II: Mechanism of Action - How Food Sensitivities May Cause Skin Conditions — 41

CHAPTER 3: Immune System Response and Food Sensitivities — 43

   Inflammation — 43
   Mediators of Inflammation: Cytokines — 44
   Mediators of Inflammation: Prostaglandins — 47
   Mediators of Inflammation: Leukotrienes — 50

CHAPTER 4: Histamine and Food Sensitivities — 53

   All About Histamine — 53
   Mast Cell Activation Syndrome (MCAS) — 58
   Histamine Intolerance (HIT) — 62
   Key Differences Between MCAS and HIT — 64

CHAPTER 5: Gut-Skin Axis and Food Sensitivities — 65

   Definitions: Leaky Gut, Gut Microbiome, and Gut Inflammation — 65
   Causes of Leaky Gut: Poor Diet — 69
   Causes of Leaky Gut: Nonsteroidal Anti-Inflammatory Drugs (NSAIDs) — 72
   Causes of Leaky Gut: Antibiotics — 74
   Causes of Leaky Gut: Proton Pump Inhibitors (PPIs) — 76
   Causes of Leaky Gut: Chronic Stress — 78
   Causes of Leaky Gut: Infections — 80
   Leaky Gut and Various Medical Conditions — 81
   Gastrointestinal Diseases — 81
   Autoimmune Diseases — 83
   Mental Health — 84
   Leaky Gut and Food Sensitivities: Bidirectional Relationship — 87
   Acne And Leaky Gut — 89
   Eczema and Psoriasis and Leaky Gut — 90
   Rosacea and Leaky Gut — 91
   Nutrient Deficiencies in Leaky Gut and their Skin Manifestations — 92
   Diagnosing Leaky Gut — 93

CHAPTER 6: Hormones and Food Sensitivities — 97

   Insulin and Insulin-Like Growth Factor (IGF-1) and Skin Health — 97
   Androgens: Testosterone and Dihydrotestosterone (DHT) and Skin Health — 98
   Estrogen and Skin Health — 100

Progesterone and Skin Health … 105
Thyroid Hormones and Skin Health … 107
Cortisol and Skin Health … 111

PART III: Common Food Sensitivities and Their Skin Effects … 115

CHAPTER 7: Gluten Sensitivity and Skin Conditions … 117

Gliadin … 117
Celiac Disease … 118
Gluten Sensitivity … 121
Wheat Sensitivity … 122
Managing Gluten Sensitivity … 125
Common Nutrient Deficiencies When Going Gluten-Free … 126

CHAPTER 8: Dairy Sensitivity and Skin Conditions … 129

Dairy Allergy … 130
Lactose Intolerance … 130
Dairy Sensitivity … 133
Managing Dairy Sensitivity … 135

CHAPTER 9: Soy Sensitivity and Skin Conditions … 137

Phytoestrogens in Soy and Hormonal Disruption … 137
Soy and Thyroid Function … 138
How Soy May Affect Your Skin … 139
Managing Soy Sensitivity … 140

CHAPTER 10: Sugar Sensitivity and Skin Conditions … 141

Skin Diseases and Sugar … 142
Aging and Sugar (Glycation) … 145
Telomere Length and Sugar … 147
Skin Infections and Sugar … 147
Hyperpigmentation and Sugar … 148
Managing Sugar Sensitivity … 150
Beware of Sugar Substitutes … 151

CHAPTER 11: Egg Sensitivity and Skin Conditions — 153

- Facts About Eggs — 153
- Skin Diseases and Eggs — 155
- Cross-Reactivity Between Egg Allergies and Flu Vaccines — 155
- Managing Egg Sensitivity — 156

CHAPTER 12: Nuts and Seeds Sensitivity and Skin Conditions — 159

- Facts About Nuts and Seeds — 159
- Cross-Reactivity: Pollen-Food Syndrome or Oral Allergy Syndrome (OAS) — 161
- Managing Nuts and Seeds Sensitivity — 163

CHAPTER 13: Caffeine Sensitivity and Skin Conditions — 165

- Mechanism of Caffeine Sensitivity — 166
- Genetics of Caffeine Sensitivity — 166
- Skin Diseases and Caffeine — 168
- Managing Caffeine Sensitivity — 170
- Caffeine-Containing Medications — 172

CHAPTER 14: Wine Sensitivity and Skin Conditions — 173

- Components of Wine: Histamines — 173
- Components of Wine: Sulfites — 174
- Components of Wine: Tannins and Flavonoids — 174
- Components of Wine: Alcohol — 175
- Skin Diseases And Wine — 177
- Managing Wine Sensitivity — 178

CHAPTER 15: Chocolate Sensitivity and Skin Conditions — 181

- Components of Chocolate — 181
- Skin Diseases and Chocolate — 183
- Managing Chocolate Sensitivity — 184

CHAPTER 16: FODMAP Sensitivity and Skin Conditions — 185

- Definitions of FODMAPS — 185
- Skin Diseases and Fodmaps — 188
- Managing FODMAP Sensitivity — 188

CHAPTER 17: Shellfish Sensitivity and Skin Conditions — 191

    Components of Shellfish — 191
    Skin Diseases and Shellfish — 192
    Managing Shellfish Sensitivity — 193

CHAPTER 18: Nightshade Vegetables Sensitivity and Skin Conditions — 195

    Components of Nightshades — 195
    Skin Diseases and Nightshades — 197
    Managing Nightshade Sensitivity — 197

PART IV: Identifying Food Sensitivities — **199**

CHAPTER 19: Food Diary — 201

CHAPTER 20: Elimination Diet — 203

    Phases of Elimination Diet — 204
    The Negatives of Elimination Diet — 206

CHAPTER 21: Testing for Food Sensitivities — 209

    2 Types of Food Sensitivity Tests — 211
    IgG-Based Food Sensitivities Testing — 211
    Clinical Considerations in IgG Testing — 215
    Non-IgG Based Food Sensitivity Testing — 216
    Comparison of Food Sensitivity Tests — 222

PART V: The Clear Skin Diet and Lifestyle Recommendations — **227**

CHAPTER 22: Clear Skin Diet — 229

    Whole Foods — 230
    Fiber — 231
    Macronutrients: Carbohydrates — 235
    Macronutrients: Proteins — 235
    Plant-Based Proteins — 236
    Animal-Based Proteins — 238
    Macronutrients: Fats — 239
    Herbs and Spices — 241
    Nuts and Seeds — 242

Water	245
Probiotics	250
Prebiotics	255
Glutamine	258
Collagen	261
Omega-3 Fatty Acids	263
CHAPTER 23: Clear Skin Lifestyle	267
Mindful Eating	268
Examples of Stress-Reducing Activities	270
The Importance of Good Sleep	271
Exercise	273
Positive and Meaningful Connections	274
CONCLUSION	**277**
REFERENCES	**281**
About the Author	**300**

INTRODUCTION

In today's world, our skin is often seen as a reflection of our overall health and well-being. We spend insane amounts of resources on skincare products, treatments, and procedures to achieve that coveted, flawless complexion. Yet, despite our best efforts, many of us still struggle with persistent skin issues such as acne, eczema, psoriasis, and other dermatological conditions. What if the solution lies not just in what we apply to our skin but also in what we consume?

"The Clear Skin Diet: Unlocking the Secret Link Between Food Sensitivities and Skin Health" explores the often-overlooked connection between diet and skin health. While the skincare industry emphasizes topical treatments, more data show that the foods we eat can significantly impact our skin condition. In this book, you will learn how to discover your hidden food sensitivities and implement the components of the Clear Skin Diet that apply to you. Based on that, we will provide detailed advice on adjusting your diet, suggest beneficial foods to incorporate, and recommend supplements that help with nutritional deficiencies.

// INTRODUCTION

Who is this book for?

This book is for anybody interested in how their body functions! Whether you have a skin issue or not, finding out how our health directly reflects the foods we eat is fascinating. The appearance of our skin is often just the tip of the iceberg, signaling to us what is going on deep underneath.

This book is focused on skin and expresses my two passions: skin health and functional medicine. Functional medicine is a personalized medical approach that offers natural, whole-body care and addresses the root causes of diseases.

I am a Western-trained MD and a certified functional medicine provider, which can make me either divided or more rounded. I hope that the latter is the case!

At our skin clinic, we treat various skin conditions utilizing both conventional and functional medicine philosophies. Of course, a combination of both approaches is ideal. Yet, the functional medicine approach may be time-consuming, expensive, and difficult for some because it is usually not a quick fix. It requires a patient to be a full-fledged partner in their treatment plan rather than a medical care receiver. Respect for the patient's preferences is the key to our approach. For example, while conventional medicine offers a steroid cream to make the eczema flare-up go away, functional medicine aims to look at every aspect of the patient's well-being, such as diet, stress, exposure to toxins, exercise routine, in-depth family and childhood history, major triggering events in life and more to get to the cause of eczema. All these factors make one who they are, and everybody's story is different.

In writing this book, my goal was to make it concise, avoid repetitions as much as possible, and make it easy to use. In my years of counseling patients about their health, I have learned to avoid big terms of "medicalese" that may sound scary and confusing. This book is written in simple and easy-to-understand language to make it accessible to anybody without any medical or scientific background. Simple and colorful images and graphics make some science concepts more fun.

Although I focus on food sensitivities as potential causes of skin conditions, they can't be solely blamed for all skin conditions. There are many other factors and influences, such as the impact of everyday toxins, such as the ones in our skin creams and makeup. Yet, the impact of food is fundamental, and that is why I chose to focus on that.

Unlike immediate allergic reactions, food sensitivities can produce subtle, chronic symptoms that are easy to overlook. These sensitivities can lead to systemic inflammation, hormonal imbalances, and disruptions in gut health—all of which can manifest visibly on our skin.

The book will help you identify common food triggers, such as gluten, dairy, soy, sugar, eggs, FODMAPs, nightshades, shellfish, wine, chocolate, caffeine, nuts, and seeds, and their specific impact on various skin conditions.

The Clear Skin Diet is not dogmatic; it is a template that you can easily use and personalize. We are all different with our unique

// INTRODUCTION

set of genes and unique life experiences, including our environment, stressors, toxins, and lifestyle habits. All these factors make us who we are, so one diet can't be applied to everybody.

Personalization is the key concept in functional medicine. It means you need to know yourself and your body before starting a specific food plan.

Ultimately, this book is about more than just achieving clear skin.

It is also about understanding and listening to your body, recognizing the interconnectedness of diet and health, and taking steps towards a healthier version of yourself.

It means that as you work on improving your skin by following particular dietary recommendations and cutting out foods you are sensitive to, you may notice that your migraine is gone, your joints no longer ache, and your brain fog has lifted. I see this transformational power of food all the time in our clinic.

By the end of this journey, you will have the knowledge and tools to manage your food sensitivities and cultivate a harmonious relationship between your diet and your skin.

Here is the outline of this book:

It starts by discussing how food sensitivities differ from food allergies in their immune mechanism, manifestations, duration, etc.

One of the most empowering aspects of managing food sensitivities is the control it gives you over your health. By addressing our whole well-being, we can mitigate our food sensitivities and, in some cases, eliminate them. That is the crucial point of that chapter.

Then, we will explore how food sensitivities work: what they do to our body and skin, particularly to cause symptoms. Lightly, we will go into the foundations of immune system and its mediators, such as cytokines, prostaglandins, leukotrienes, and histamine. We will focus on the latter by discussing mast cell activation syndrome and histamine intolerance.

Then, we will move on to the concepts of leaky gut and gut dysbiosis that are becoming more accepted in conventional medicine. There is now abundant research connecting gut health to almost every organ in our body, with gut dysfunction causing a variety of issues, from irritable bowel syndrome to eczema to neurodegenerative diseases like Alzheimer's and Parkinson's disease.

Next, we will focus on our hormones, such as insulin, testosterone, estrogen, progesterone, and cortisol, and how food sensitivities can lead to their imbalance.

We will then move on to the heart of the book, which goes over common food sensitivities, such as gluten, eggs, dairy, etc., and how and why they affect our skin. Skin is the largest organ in our body and doesn't exist in isolation. It functions as a mirror to our general health, so we will touch upon the common detrimental effects of these trigger foods on our whole body. For example, did you know that for some people, drinking more than 3-4 cups of coffee per day may lead to non-fatal heart attacks? As a coffee lover, it breaks my heart, too!

// INTRODUCTION

Each chapter in this section discusses how trigger foods affect our skin and lists obvious and hidden sources of the trigger components in everyday foods. For example, did you know gluten is often found in soy sauce?

The following section will address one of the most common questions asked at our clinic: "How do I find out what I am sensitive to?" That is the crux of the matter, isn't it? Often, patients start listing a variety of symptoms, both skin and non-skin-related, trying to guess at connections between foods and these symptoms. So, in this section, we will go over how you can discover your food sensitivities in an organized fashion. We will discuss in detail the food sensitivity testing, what it entails, and how it is done while providing a sample report that includes testing of 176 foods.

Finally, we will reach the culmination of this book by providing a template for a Clear Skin Diet. In this key chapter of the book, we will focus on foods, vitamins, and supplements at the heart of a healthy diet. This template is gut, immune, and hormone-health-friendly. Incorporating it with your specific food sensitivity recommendations will help your personalized plan.

Of course, I strongly recommend discussing any changes in your diet with your healthcare provider and a nutritionist. The key to every diet is that it must be personalized. While many of the food concepts in this book fundamentally benefit almost everyone, the diet, and supplements must be adjusted if you have diabetes, kidney disease, or recent intestinal surgery: each condition will require further personalization. So, please have your professional medical team help you with the positive changes that you are about to embark on.

Welcome to "The Clear Skin Diet: Unlocking the Secret Link Between Food Sensitivities and Skin Health!"

PART I

Food Sensitivities and Skin Health

Definitions and Key Concepts

CHAPTER 1

Understanding Food Sensitivities

How They Differ from Food Allergies

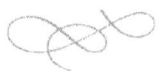

While food allergies are widely recognized and understood, with their dramatic and immediate reactions, food sensitivities present a quieter but persistent challenge. They can lead to chronic skin conditions and other health issues that aren't as easily traced back to a specific food. By shining a light on these silent triggers, this book can help you uncover the hidden culprits behind your skin woes and guide you toward the path of luminous skin.

In this chapter, we will examine the differences between these two conditions, specifically focusing on their immunology, onset, diagnosis, longevity, half-life, and food amounts needed to elicit a reaction.

Food Sensitivities vs. Food Allergies: The Overview

Food Sensitivities

Food sensitivities are often compared to slow-developing storms, as they may often take hours or even days to show symptoms. Due to delayed symptoms, identifying the specific cause or a specific food can be challenging.

These symptoms could present as gastrointestinal reactions such as bloating, gassy sensation, and abdominal pain. In addition to abdominal discomfort, food sensitivities can lead to systemic effects such as headaches, fatigue, and joint pain. Furthermore, they can worsen chronic skin conditions, including eczema, acne, and rosacea. Over time, these persistent symptoms can significantly impact your quality of life, requiring careful observation and a methodical approach to identify and manage the underlying triggers.

Food Allergies

In contrast, food allergies are marked by immediate and often dramatic responses. When you eat a food, you are allergic to, your immune system reacts quickly and strongly, treating the food as a harmful substance. This can cause symptoms to appear rapidly, such as hives, swelling, itching, and digestive problems like nausea or vomiting.

The most severe allergic reactions involve the respiratory system, potentially causing difficulty breathing, wheezing, and, in extreme cases, anaphylaxis—a life-threatening condition where your whole body shuts down. Skin reactions may manifest as hives, whole body rash, or swelling of the lips, tongue, throat, or entire body.

Such reactions demand prompt attention and typically require avoiding the offending food altogether. Individuals with severe food allergies often need to carry emergency medication, such as an EpiPen, to manage accidental exposures and prevent life-threatening complications.

Food Sensitivities vs. Food Allergies: Immunology

Food Sensitivities

Food sensitivities engage a more subdued and less aggressive part of the immune system. This process is frequently mediated by Immunoglobulin G (IgG) antibodies and less commonly by Immunoglobulin A (IgA) antibodies. IgG is the most common type of antibody in the bloodstream and is primarily responsible for identifying and neutralizing pathogens.

A pathogen is anything that our body considers hostile. Usually, pathogens are harmful bacteria, viruses, parasites, fungi, and toxins. However, in the case of food sensitivities, these antibodies can mistake certain foods as harmful, leading to an ongoing, low-level immune response.

In some cases, this reaction might not be immune-mediated but can result from enzyme deficiencies or other non-immune mechanisms, causing a slower, prolonged response. Imagine a pot simmering on the stove: the heat is low, and it takes a while before it starts bubbling and boiling.

Food Allergies

In stark contrast, food allergies trigger a rapid and intense immune response. This reaction is typically mediated by Immunoglobulin E (IgE), which is specifically designed to combat parasites but can mistakenly target certain foods. When a person with a food allergy consumes the allergen, their body quickly produces IgEs, which bind to it. This triggers other immune cells to start releasing histamines and other chemicals.

This process happens at the lightning speed, causing an immediate and often severe reaction. It's like a fire alarm going off when smoke is detected: the body goes into a heightened state of alert, and symptoms such as hives, swelling, difficulty breathing, and anaphylaxis can occur within minutes. This swift and aggressive response is how the immune system protects the body from what it perceives as a dangerous invader, even though the food itself is harmless to most people.

Food Sensitivities vs. Food Allergies: Onset

Food Sensitivities

The onset of symptoms due to food sensitivities is like a slow-burning mystery novel where the plot unfolds gradually. After consuming the offending food, symptoms can appear between 2 to 72 hours. This delayed reaction complicates identifying the specific trigger, requiring meticulous detective work and a keen eye for patterns. Imagine eating a meal on Monday and only experiencing discomfort on Wednesday; the connection between the food and the symptoms isn't immediately obvious.

Food Allergies

In contrast, the onset of symptoms from food allergies resembles a high-stakes thriller where the villain is caught red-handed. Symptoms typically occur within minutes to a couple of hours after consuming the allergen, making it much easier to identify the trigger. This immediate reaction is like a flashing neon sign pointing to the culprit. For instance, someone might eat a peanut cookie and almost instantly experience hives, swelling, or difficulty breathing.

This rapid onset of symptoms can range from mild to severe and life-threatening, such as anaphylaxis. The swift and dramatic nature of allergic reactions makes it straightforward for individuals to pinpoint which foods to avoid. Most people with food allergies are acutely aware of their triggers and take precautions to prevent exposure.

Food Sensitivities vs. Food Allergies: Diagnosis

Food Sensitivities

Identifying food sensitivities could be frustrating for both the patient and the provider. The delayed onset of symptoms means that the offending food might not be immediately apparent, requiring a thorough and meticulous approach to diagnosis.

How are food sensitivities diagnosed?

Common methods used to pinpoint food sensitivities include maintaining a food diary and following an elimination diet. A food diary involves keeping a detailed record of everything you eat and noting any symptoms that arise. It can help identify patterns and potential triggers. An elimination diet involves removing suspected foods from your diet for a period and then gradually reintroducing them one at a time to observe if symptoms reappear. These methods can be effective in identifying specific food sensitivities and managing associated symptoms.

Additionally, there are now several food sensitivity laboratory tests that utilize different techniques. Some commercial labs measure IgG antibodies to specific foods, others assess the reaction of the white blood cells to the same triggers. The main distinction is that the first method focuses on immunoglobulins and the other on the level of inflammation in the whole blood. Both techniques are acceptable methods of diagnosing food sensitivities. We will discuss the diagnosis of food sensitivities in more detail in *Chapter 21. Testing for Food Sensitivities.*

Food Allergies

Diagnosing food allergies is typically more straightforward due to the immediate and obvious nature of the reactions. Here are some common methods used to diagnose and/or confirm food allergies:

Skin Prick Test

A skin prick test is common for diagnosing allergies to various substances, such as foods, pollen, pet dander, and dust mites. The test is usually conducted on the forearm or upper back, where the skin is relatively smooth and easy to work with.

The testing area is sterilized with alcohol. Small drops of potential allergens are placed on the skin. These allergens can be a wide range of substances, including specific foods, pollens, animal dander, mold spores, and dust mites. A small, sterile lancet is used to prick the skin through each drop of allergen. This allows a tiny amount of the allergen to enter just below the surface of the skin. The pricking is shallow and generally not painful, although it may cause minor discomfort. The patient waits about 15 to 20 minutes to allow any reactions to develop. During this time, the healthcare provider will observe the skin for any signs of a reaction. If the patient is allergic to a substance, a raised, red, itchy bump (like a bug bite) will appear at the site of the prick. This is known as wheal.

The size of the wheal is measured to determine the severity of the reaction. Larger wheals generally indicate a stronger allergic response.

The skin prick test is quick and efficient with minimal discomfort. It is quite comprehensive, and less expensive than blood tests.

However, skin prick tests may not always be accurate. Factors such as skin conditions, medications, and the tester's skill can influence results. Also, they are not suitable for all patients: patients with certain skin conditions (like eczema) at the time of testing (a patch of normal skin is needed) or those who are at high risk for severe allergic reactions (anaphylaxis) may not be suitable candidates for skin prick testing.

Blood Test

Measuring the levels of specific IgE immunoglobulins in the blood can help identify allergies to particular foods.

Blood allergy tests, also known as specific IgE blood tests or radioallergosorbent tests (RAST), are used to detect allergic responses to particular substances by measuring specific antibodies in the blood. During this test, the blood sample is analyzed at the lab by being exposed to various allergens, which can include foods, pollen, pet dander, dust mites, mold, and other common triggers. The levels of IgEs that bind to each allergen are measured.

The higher levels of specific IgE antibodies indicate a potential allergic reaction to the corresponding allergen. These results are usually quantified, providing a numerical value that helps determine the severity of the sensitivity. The positive aspect of the blood allergy tests is that, unlike skin prick tests, the blood tests are safe for individuals with skin conditions, those at risk of severe allergic reactions, or those who cannot discontinue certain medications. The downside of the blood allergy tests is that they could be less sensitive, producing both false- positive and false-negative results. Also, they may take some time, from days to weeks.

Oral Food Challenge (OFC)

Oral Food Challenge is considered the standard for diagnosing allergies. During this test, under medical supervision small amounts of the suspected allergen are consumed to monitor for a reaction.

The procedure is conducted under the supervision of an allergist or a trained medical professional in a medical setting, such as a hospital, where emergency treatment can be administered if needed. Patients are usually asked to avoid antihistamines or other allergy medications that could affect the test results for a specified period before the challenge. The food is initially administered in small doses, which are slowly increased at regular intervals. Meanwhile, the patient is closely monitored for any allergic reactions, including hives, swelling, stomach pain, vomiting, wheezing, or anaphylaxis.

If a reaction occurs, the challenge is stopped immediately, and appropriate treatment is provided. After the final dose, the patient remains under observation for an additional period (usually a few hours) to ensure no delayed reactions occur. The allergist evaluates and discusses the results with the patient, providing guidance on managing the allergy if a reaction was observed or confirming the absence of an allergy if no reaction occurred.

The benefit of the OFC is that it provides clear and definitive evidence of whether a person is allergic to a specific food, eliminating uncertainties that might arise from other testing methods. Additionally, it helps identify the exact threshold at which a person can tolerate a food, providing detailed information on the severity of the allergy. A negative OFC can expand a patient's diet, improving their quality of life by allowing them to safely include foods they previously avoided. Finally, confirming or ruling out an allergy can significantly reduce anxiety for patients and their families, providing peace of mind and clear guidelines for dietary choices.

The primary risk of an OFC is the possible onset of a life-threatening reaction. However, conducting the test in a controlled medical setting minimizes this risk. Additionally, this testing process can be lengthy, requiring a significant time commitment from the patient and the medical staff.

Food Sensitivities vs. Food Allergies: Longevity

Food Sensitivities

One of the distinguishing features of food sensitivities is their potential to diminish or even disappear over time. For instance, you may be sensitized to melons and react to them with a mild rash. By avoiding melons for a period and perhaps reintroducing them gradually, you may find that your sensitivity to melons lessens or completely resolves.

Several factors contribute to this potential for resolution:

- ❖ *Gut Health Improvement*: Enhancing gut health through probiotics, prebiotics, and a balanced diet can often alleviate food sensitivities. A healthier gut microbiome can improve the body's tolerance of certain foods. More about that in *Chapter 21. Clear Skin Diet*
- ❖ *Enzyme Supplementation*: For sensitivities related to enzyme deficiencies, enzyme supplements can help the body digest these foods better, potentially reducing or eliminating symptoms over time.
- ❖ *Changes in the Immune System*: Sensitivities may lessen as the immune system becomes less reactive, possibly through improved overall health and reduced exposure to triggers.

Food sensitivities are less daunting than food allergies because of their flexibility and potential for change. With the right approach and time, many people find that their sensitivities can be managed or even outgrown, allowing for a more varied diet without discomfort.

Food Allergies

In contrast, food allergies tend to be more persistent and long-lasting. While some children may outgrow specific allergies (like milk or egg allergies), many food allergies, particularly those to nuts, shellfish, and fish, are likely to persist for life. This longevity is due to the nature of the immune response involved in allergies, which is typically lifelong and can become more severe with repeated exposures.

The reasons food allergies rarely go away include:

- *Immune Memory*: The immune system's memory of the allergen remains robust, continuing to produce IgE antibodies and causing reactions upon exposure.
- *Lack of Desensitization*: Unlike food sensitivities, where gradual reintroduction might be possible, food allergies require strict avoidance. This constant vigilance means the immune system never has a chance to become desensitized to the allergen.
- *Severity of Reactions:* The potential for severe, life-threatening reactions such as anaphylaxis necessitates ongoing avoidance and readiness to respond to accidental exposures with medications like antihistamines and epinephrine.

While ongoing research efforts and experimental treatments aim to desensitize individuals to certain food allergens, these are not yet widely available or guaranteed to be effective. As a result, most people with food allergies must maintain lifelong avoidance of their specific triggers.

Food Sensitivities vs. Food Allergies: Half-Life

Let's simplify the concept of half-life with a relatable example. Imagine you have a pile of cookies and eat half of what's left every hour. If you start with 16 cookies, you'll have 8 cookies after one hour. After the next hour, you'll have 4 cookies, then 2, and so on. This repetitive process of halving the cookies each time is like a half-life.

In scientific terms, the half-life is the time it takes for half of a substance to break down or be eliminated from your body.

Food Sensitivities

IgG antibodies, the principal antibodies in food sensitivities, have a relatively long half-life of around 21 days. This means that every 21 days, half of the IgG antibodies are broken down and removed from your system.

So, if you start with 100 IgG antibodies, then after 21 days, you'll have 50 left. Another 21 days later, you'll have 25, and so on.

Due to a longer half-life, food sensitivities can linger for longer durations.

It may now make sense why the recommended duration for an elimination diet should be at least three weeks, as after 21 days, the amount of IgG antibodies to trigger foods will be halved.

Food Allergies

IgE antibodies, associated with immediate allergic reactions, have a half-life of about 2.3 days. That is why food allergies don't stick around in the body for very long. When you have a food allergy, these IgE antibodies react quickly to certain foods, causing symptoms like hives, swelling, or even anaphylaxis right after eating the allergen.

The difference in the half-life of IgE and IgG antibodies can help distinguish between food allergies and sensitivities.

Food Sensitivities vs. Food Allergies: Food Amounts Needed to Elicit a Reaction

Food Sensitivities

Food sensitivities are portion dependent. For example, you might be able to enjoy a small serving of a certain food without any problems, but if you eat a larger portion, you might start to feel uncomfortable with symptoms like rash, bloating, headaches, or fatigue.

Food Allergies

With food allergies, even a tiny bit of the offending food can trigger a reaction. This is because IgE antibodies get activated the same way, regardless of the amount of food ingested. It is an all-or-nothing reaction!

To sum up, recognizing the difference between food sensitivities and food allergies is crucial for effective management and treatment. Mislabeling someone with a food allergy when they actually have food sensitivity can lead to unnecessary dietary restrictions and anxiety. While food allergies require immediate medical intervention and avoidance of the allergen, managing food sensitivities often involves a more nuanced approach, like keeping a food diary, undergoing elimination diets and food testing, and seeking guidance from healthcare professionals.

CHAPTER 2

Definitions of Skin Conditions Linked to Food Sensitivities

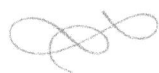

Before exploring common foods that trigger various skin conditions, let's review the definitions of these conditions. This list is not all-inclusive, as one may argue that all skin conditions are related to the foods that we eat in one way or another. Yet this list represents common skin diseases that are known to be triggered or worsened by certain foods in people with food sensitivities.

Acne

Acne is characterized by the inflammation of hair follicles and sebaceous (oil) glands, leading to various skin manifestations. These manifestations include pimples, blackheads, whiteheads, cysts, and nodules.

Sebum is the oily substance produced by sebaceous glands in the skin epidermis. It is composed mainly of triglycerides, free fatty acids, wax esters, squalene, and cholesterol. Sebum lubricates and protects the skin, but too much sebum can clog pores, leading to acne development.

Acne begins when hair follicles become clogged and obstructed with dead skin cells and sebum, creating an environment favorable for bacterial growth. The blocked follicles provide a habitat for bacteria, particularly *Cutibacterium acnes* (formerly *Propionibacterium acnes*), which can cause inflammation and infection.

Acne primarily affects areas with a high prevalence of sebum-producing glands, such as the face, scalp, chest, back, shoulders, and upper arms.

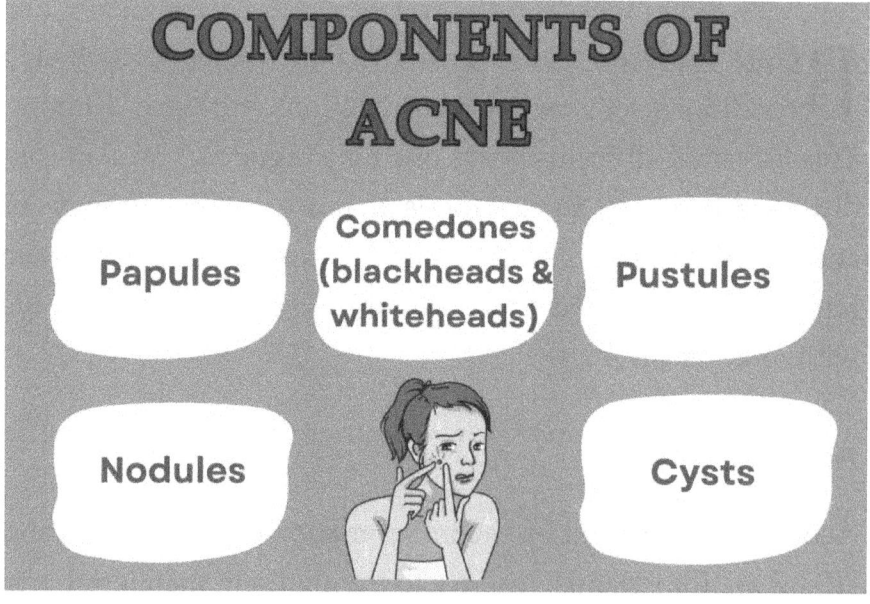

Figure 2.1. Components of Acne.

Non-Food Related Factors Predisposing to Acne

❖ *Hormonal Changes:* Hormonal fluctuations, especially during puberty, menstruation, pregnancy, and stress, can increase sebum production, leading to acne.

- ❖ *Genetics*: A family history of acne is a predisposing factor.
- ❖ *Stress*: Psychological stress can trigger or worsen acne outbreaks.

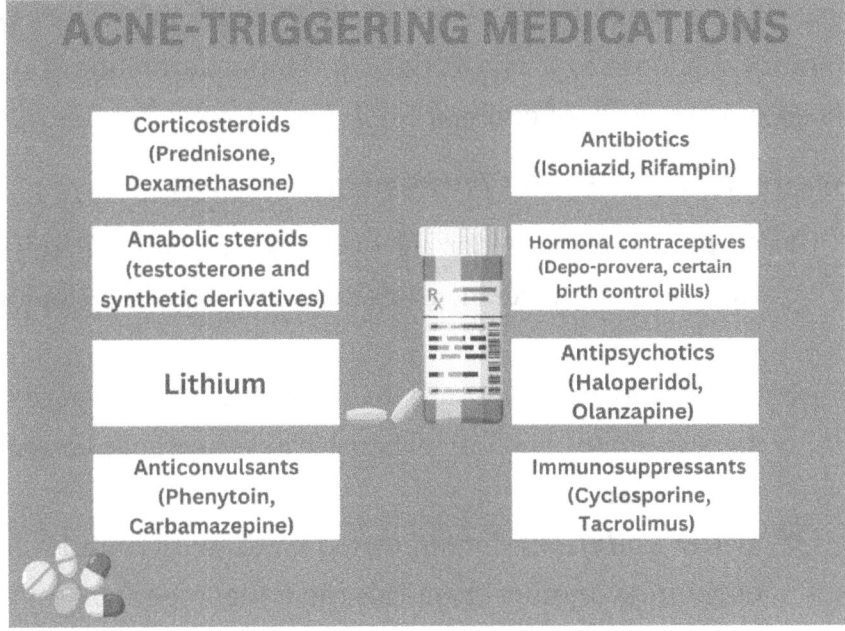

Figure 2.2 Acne-triggering Medications.

Eczema

Eczema is a long-lasting skin condition with itchy, dry, and inflamed patches. It is often seen in children but can affect people of all ages.

In eczema the skin becomes very dry, red, inflamed and more sensitive to irritants and allergens. Patches of eczema can appear on various body parts, including the face, neck, hands, feet, and the insides of elbows and knees.

In more severe cases, the skin may ooze fluid and form crusts.

Chronic itching is a hallmark of eczema and can be worse at night. Chronic scratching can cause the skin to thicken, leading to a leathery texture.

One of the main mechanisms of eczema is an overactive immune response to various triggers. Atopic dermatitis is the most common form of eczema.

Non-Food Related Factors Predisposing to Eczema

- *Genetic Factors*: A family history of eczema, allergies, asthma, or hay fever increases the likelihood of developing eczema.
- *Air Pollution:* Exposure to pollutants such cigarette smoke, smog, and car exhaust can exacerbate eczema symptoms.
- *Water Pollution:* Contaminated water with high levels of chlorine or other chemicals can irritate the skin.
- *Irritants*: Soaps, detergents, shampoos, disinfectants, and juices from fruits or vegetables.
- *Wool and Synthetic Fabrics*: Rough, scratchy fabrics like wool and certain synthetics
- *Tight Clothing*: Wearing tight clothing can cause friction and sweating, leading to eczema symptoms.
- *Allergens:* Dust mites, pet dander, pollen, mold, and foods.
- *Climate:* Extreme temperatures, high or low humidity, and sweating.
- *Stress*: Emotional stress can worsen eczema symptoms.

Seborrheic Dermatitis

Seborrheic dermatitis is a type of eczema. Similarly to acne, seborrheic dermatitis affects areas abundant in sebaceous glands, such as the scalp and face, and less so the upper chest. However, unlike acne, it has a higher affinity for the scalp. It manifests as red, greasy, and flaky patches, often with yellow or white scales. This condition manifests as dandruff of the face and scalp. Cradle cap is the term for seborrheic dermatitis in infants.

The yeast Malassezia is believed to be a key player in the development of seborrheic dermatitis. Various factors, including stress, cold and dry weather, and hormonal changes, can exacerbate symptoms.

Contact Dermatitis

Contact dermatitis is characterized by skin inflammation following exposure to a specific substance. It has 2 subtypes:

- *Irritant Contact Dermatitis*: This happens when something directly irritates the skin, like soap, detergent, or a harsh chemical. It can cause skin to become dry, cracked, and sore.
- *Allergic Contact Dermatitis*: This occurs when your skin has an immune reaction to a substance. Common allergens include latex, poison ivy, certain metals like nickel, and some fragrances or cosmetics. The reaction can cause a red, itchy rash that might develop blisters.

In both cases, the affected skin area can feel uncomfortable, and the symptoms usually appear shortly after contact with the irritating substance. The best way to treat contact dermatitis is to avoid the substance that causes the reaction.

Psoriasis

Psoriasis is a condition in which the immune system attacks healthy skin cells due to an autoimmune response, speeding up their production and forming plaques.

Psoriasis is a skin condition resulting from an altered autoimmune response, marked by the accelerated growth and accumulation of skin cells, forming thick, silvery, scaly patches on the skin's surface. It is often chronic, with the severity of psoriasis ranging from mild and limited to a few areas on the body to severe and diffuse, covering most of the body. The common areas affected by psoriasis are elbows, knees, scalp, and lower back. Psoriasis may also affect the nails, causing color changes and nail deformity. It is a non-contagious condition with periods of remission and flare-ups.

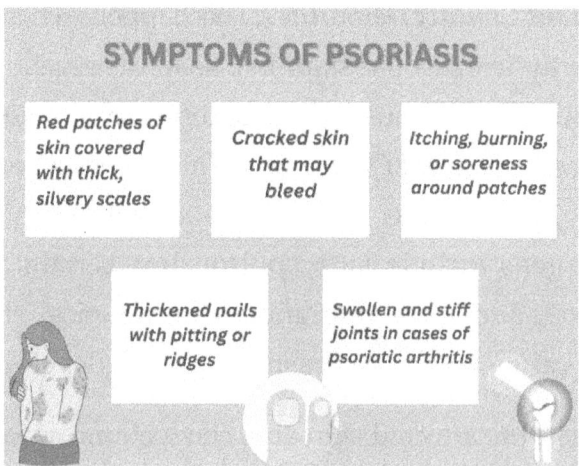

Figure 2.3 Symptoms of psoriasis.

Non-Food Related Factors Predisposing to Psoriasis

- ❖ **Genetic Factors**: Several genes have been found to predispose to psoriasis.
- ❖ **Infections**: Streptococcal throat infections can trigger a form of psoriasis called guttate psoriasis.
- ❖ **Injury to the Skin**: Cuts, scrapes, insect bites, or sunburn can cause a psoriasis flare-up, a phenomenon known as the Koebner response.
- ❖ **Weather**: Cold, dry weather can worsen psoriasis, while sunlight may improve it.
- ❖ **Stress:** As in most skin conditions, stress is an important trigger for psoriasis, as well.

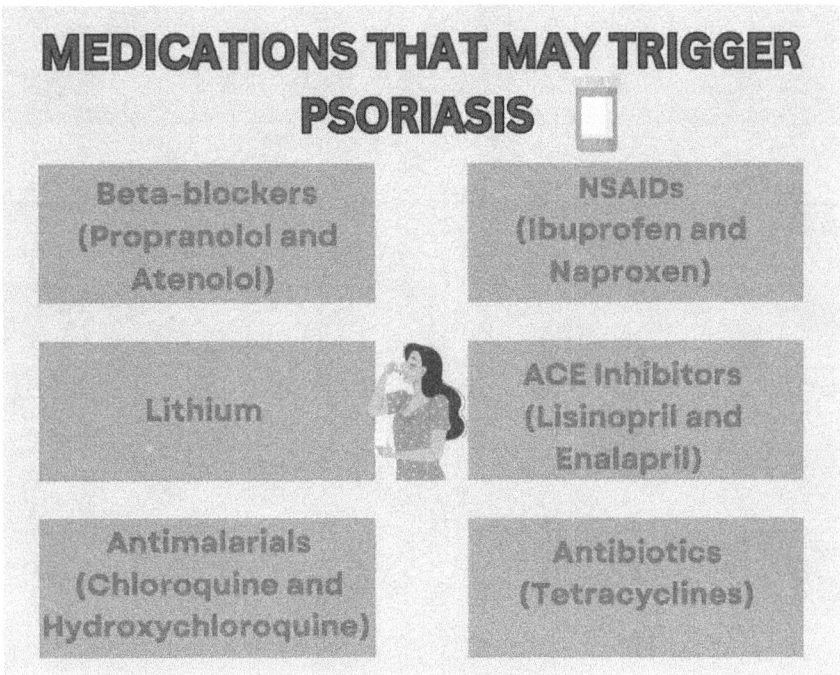

Figure 2.4 Medications that may trigger psoriasis.

Rosacea

Rosacea is a long-lasting skin condition that causes redness and sometimes small, pus-filled bumps on the face. It commonly presents with redness, visible blood vessels, swelling, and acne-like breakouts. Rosacea usually affects the central part of the face, including the cheeks, nose, forehead, and chin. It can also affect the eyes, leading to ocular rosacea. Rosacea is most common in adults aged 30 to 50 and tends to affect individuals with fair skin. Abnormality in immune system response is a major contributor to inflammation and symptoms of rosacea.

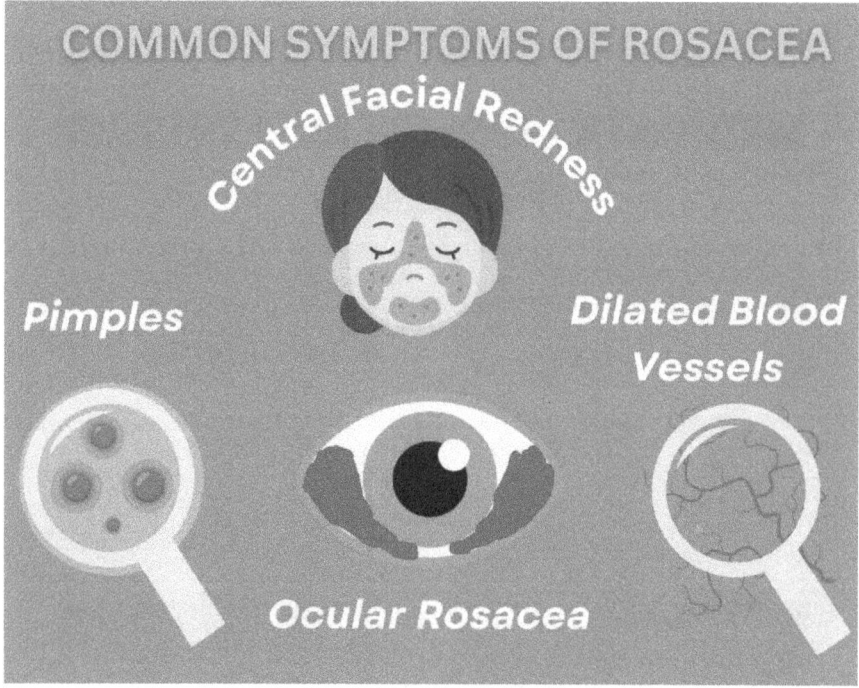

Figure 2.5 Common symptoms of rosacea.

Non-Food Related Factors Predisposing to Rosacea

- ❖ *Genetic Factors*: Rosacea has a genetic predisposition.
- ❖ *Vascular Abnormalities:* Issues with blood vessels in the face, such as hyper-responsiveness or increased blood flow, can lead to persistent redness and visible blood vessels.
- ❖ *Microbial Factors:* The presence of certain microorganisms, such as *Demodex* mites and *Helicobacter pylori* bacteria, may trigger or exacerbate rosacea.
- ❖ *Sun Exposure*: Ultraviolet (UV) radiation can aggravate rosacea, so using sunscreen is essential.
- ❖ *Temperature Extremes*: Hot or cold weather, wind, and humidity can trigger flare-ups.
- ❖ *Stress:* Always a trigger!

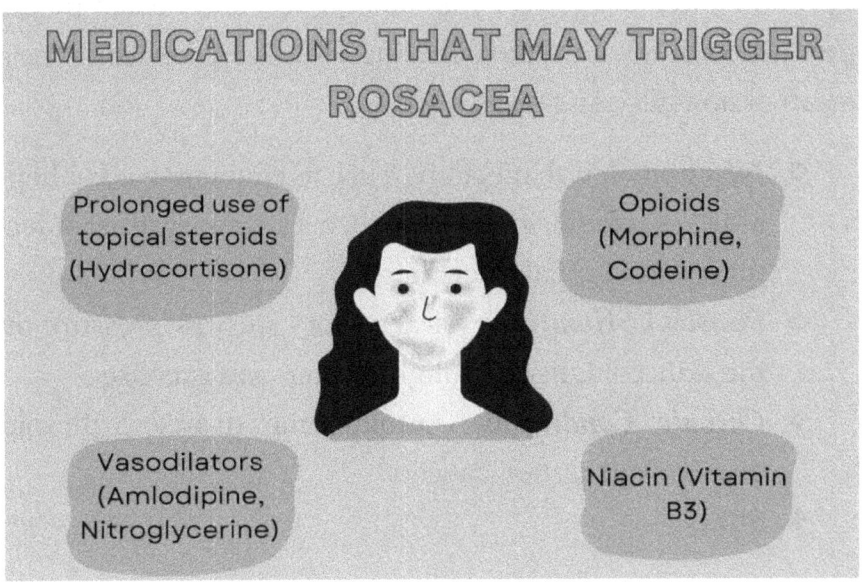

Figure 2.6 Medications that may trigger rosacea.

Hives

Hives, also known as urticaria, are a common skin reaction that manifests as the sudden appearance of raised, itchy welts (wheals) on the skin. They usually blanch (turn white) when pressed. Hives can range from small round spots to large patches, and they often change shape, move around, and appear and disappear within short periods.

Hives can be itchy and bothersome or asymptomatic. In some cases, they can cause more profound swelling of the skin, known as angioedema, particularly around the eyes, lips, hands, feet, and throat.

Non-Food Related Factors Predisposing to Hives

Hives are often triggered by an allergic reaction caused by the production of IgE immunoglobulins. However, they could be a result of non-allergic causes, such as

- *Infections:* Viral infections (such as common cold or hepatitis), bacterial infections (such as urinary tract infections), and fungal infections.
- *Physical Stimuli:* Physical factors such as pressure on the skin, cold, heat, sunlight, water, and exercise.
- *Chronic Conditions:* Autoimmune diseases, thyroid disease, and certain cancers.
- *Stress*

Types of Hives

- ❖ **Acute Urticaria** is when hives last less than six weeks.
- ❖ **Chronic Urticaria** is when hives persist for more than six weeks. The cause is often challenging to identify and may be related to an underlying health condition or autoimmune response.
- ❖ **Physical Urticaria** is urticaria triggered by physical stimuli such as pressure, temperature changes, sunlight, water, or exercise.

Physical Urticaria includes:

- ❖ **Dermatographism**: Hives that appear after the skin is scratched or rubbed.
- ❖ **Cold Urticaria**: Triggered by exposure to cold air, water, or objects.
- ❖ **Heat Urticaria**: Triggered by exposure to heat.
- ❖ **Solar Urticaria**: Triggered by exposure to sunlight.
- ❖ **Cholinergic Urticaria**: Triggered by increased body temperature from exercise, hot showers, or stress.

Latest Research

A study found that patients with urticaria have a higher risk of developing cancer compared to the general population. The risk is 49% higher in the first year following diagnosis but decreases to 6% in subsequent years. The research analyzed data from Danish healthcare databases and included 87,507 patients followed for a median of 10.1 years.

> The highest cancer risk within the first year was for hematological cancers, especially Hodgkin lymphoma.

Rashes

Rashes are noticeable changes in the skin texture, color, or appearance. They can manifest as red, inflamed areas, bumps, blotches, or scales and may occur on any body part. Rashes are a symptom rather than a specific diagnosis, resulting from various conditions and environmental factors. The severity of a rash can vary from mild irritation to severe, widespread inflammation. Rashes are a common manifestation of an allergic reaction.

Symptoms of Rashes

Most rashes are red, and redness is a sign of inflammation, representing increased blood flow to the affected areas. Rashes could be itchy or not, painful or painless. They could be limited to one area or spread all over the body. There may be accompanied blistering or swelling. Some rashes are very typical in their appearance, and their diagnosis is easy. Others may present a diagnostic challenge, necessitating a biopsy.

Non-Food Related Factors Predisposing to Rashes

- *Infections*: Many infectious diseases are characterized by rashes. Common examples include chickenpox, measles, and fungus.
- *Irritants:* Exposure to chemical irritants in soaps, detergents, cosmetics, or fabrics can cause irritant contact dermatitis, resulting in rashes.

- *Heat and Sweat:* Prolonged exposure to heat and sweating can lead to heat rash (miliaria), characterized by red, itchy bumps.
- *Medications:* Essentially, any medication can cause a rash, making it hard to find the exact culprit in somebody taking many medications.
- *Insect Bites and Stings:* Bites from mosquitoes, fleas, bedbugs, and other insects can cause localized rashes, itching, and swelling.
- *Systemic Illnesses:* Rashes can be a symptom of systemic illnesses like hepatitis, mononucleosis, Lyme disease, and some types of cancer.

Pruritus (Itching Without a Rash)

Itching without a rash, or pruritus without a rash, refers to the sensation of itching on the skin without any visible signs of irritation, redness, or other dermatological symptoms. This condition can be perplexing and uncomfortable, as the itch can be persistent and severe despite the absence of an obvious skin manifestation. In fact, I can confidently say this is one of the most frustrating complaints for the medical provider, as possibilities are endless.

Symptoms of Pruritus

The main symptom, you guessed it, is itching. It can be localized to a specific area or generalized across the body. In most cases, there are no visible signs on the skin earlier in this condition, such as rash, swelling, or bumps. However, prolonged scratching can lead to secondary symptoms like broken skin, infections, and thickened skin (lichenification).

Unfortunately, sometimes, these poor patients are not believed, or their symptoms are minimized and ignored because they are not obvious in our visually-driven society.

Non-Food Related Factors Predisposing to Pruritus

- *Dry Skin (Xerosis):* One of the most common causes, especially in older adults, is dry skin, which can lead to itching without visible rash. Cold weather, low humidity, and frequent bathing can exacerbate dry skin.
- *Liver Disease:* Liver cirrhosis or hepatitis can cause pruritus due to the accumulation of bile salts in the skin.
- *Kidney Disease:* End-stage kidney disease or chronic kidney disease can lead to uremic pruritus.
- *Thyroid Disorders:* Both high and low thyroid levels can cause itching.
- *Diabetes:* Poorly controlled diabetes can lead to dry, itchy skin.
- *Blood Disorders* include conditions like polycythemia vera and iron deficiency anemia.
- *Neurological Disorders* include multiple sclerosis and nerve damage (neuropathy)
- *Psychological Factors:* Depression and anxiety can sometimes manifest as itching in the absence of a physical cause. However, organic causes need to be excluded before coming to this conclusion.

- ❖ *Medications:* Many medications can cause pruritus as a side effect, including the medications that patient has been on for many years.
- ❖ *Hormonal Changes:* Hormonal fluctuations during pregnancy or menopause can lead to itching.

Now that we have familiarized ourselves with skin diseases to be discussed in this book, let's look at the mechanisms of how food sensitivities cause or trigger these conditions.

PART II
Mechanism of Action

How Food Sensitivities May Cause Skin Conditions

CHAPTER 3

Immune System Response and Food Sensitivities

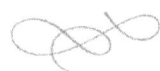

This section will explore the mechanisms by which food sensitivities affect the immune system.

This is a science portion of this book, so let's make it fun!

We will start with the concept of inflammation, which is one of the essential functions of the immune system.

Inflammation

We often speak of inflammation as a sole negative event in everyday life. We may even call somebody who is unpleasant and provoking, an "inflammatory" person. Yet, inflammation is the body's natural response to perceived threats. It is an appropriate defensive reaction of our body when danger is perceived.

Inflammation involves the release of various inflammatory mediators, including cytokines, prostaglandins, leukotrienes, histamines, and many others.

These chemicals are the messengers and executors of the immune system. When they respond appropriately to a real threat, they save us from infections and toxins from harmful microorganisms and poisonous substances. However, if for some reason, they start overreacting, we suffer in variety of ways, and our whole organism may get affected by inflammation that this overproduction creates.

Let's look at each one of them, starting with cytokines.

Mediators of Inflammation: Cytokines

Cytokines are small protein molecules. In addition to being messengers in the immune system, they are also involved in the production of blood cells. You may have heard about some types of cytokines, such as interleukins, interferons, tumor necrosis factors, and chemokines.

Interleukins are cytokines that are often named IL, followed by a number (e.g., IL-2, IL-6). Each interleukin has a specific role, such as promoting the growth of certain immune cells or triggering fever.

Cytokine storm or hypercytokinemia is when our body produces too many cytokines, leading to systemic inflammation, and in some cases organ failure and death. It may happen as a response to severe infections and some autoimmune diseases.

A subtype of cytokines called interferons can boost the immune system to fight cancer cells, and commercially produced interferon and interleukin-2 pharmaceutical agents are used to treat metastatic melanoma and kidney cancer. It is probably not surprising that while these therapies save lives, they do have many side effects, making them at times unbearable for patients.

Interestingly, there is emerging research suggesting that high levels of cytokines, such as TNF-α, Il-6, and IL-8, may be associated with anxiety and depression.

On a positive side, physical activity can increase the production of certain cytokines, which helps improve immune function and reduce inflammation. Also, cytokines are crucial in wound healing. They help attract immune cells to the wound site, promote tissue repair, and reduce infection risk.

How Cytokines May Affect Your Skin

As a broad category within the immune system, cytokines can impact the skin in various ways and may be involved in many skin disorders. Here are some of these cytokines-induced skin changes:

- *Acne:* Cytokines can stimulate sebaceous glands, leading to clogged pores.
- *Eczema:* Increased cytokine-induced inflammation may result in flare-ups.
- *Psoriasis:* Cytokines accelerate the growth cycle of skin cells, leading to the buildup of cells on the skin surface, forming thick, scaly plaques.
- *Rosacea:* Cytokine-induced chronic inflammation and vascular changes in the skin may lead to persistent redness, visible blood vessels, and sometimes pimples or pustules. Inflammation can also increase skin sensitivity and trigger flushing.

❖ *Hives:* Cytokines trigger the release of histamine from mast cells, leading to the development of hives.

Here is a graphic summary of the effects of cytokine imbalance on the skin.

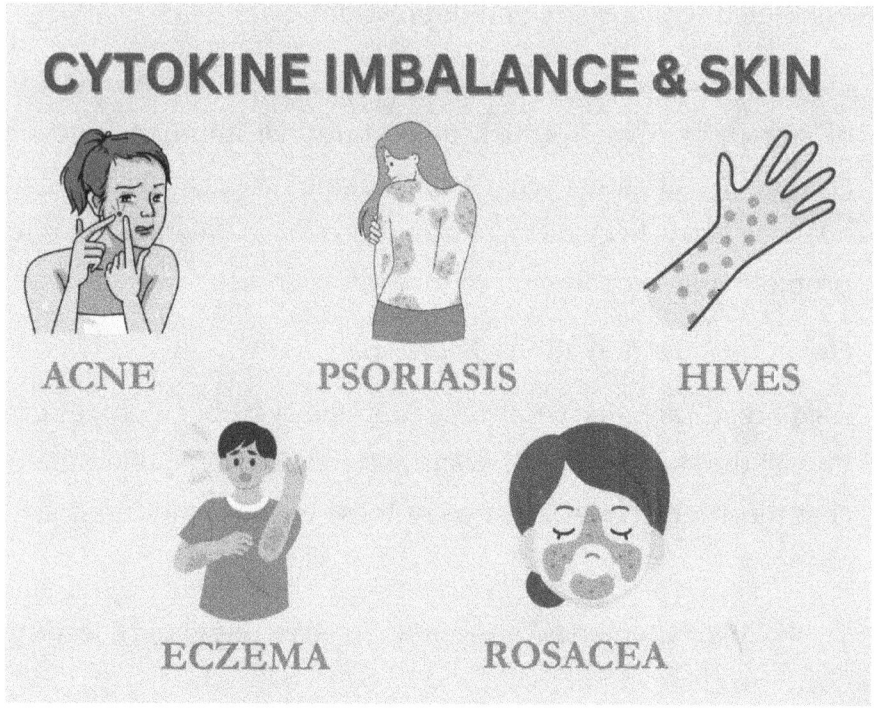

Figure 3.1 Cytokine imbalance and skin.

Let's turn our attention to the next key player in our immune system: Prostaglandins.

Mediators of Inflammation: Prostaglandins

Prostaglandins are lipid compounds that regulate inflammation and pain, control blood flow, and form blood clots. They were first discovered in the 1930s in human semen and were initially thought to come from the prostate gland, which is how they got their name. However, they are actually produced by almost all tissues in the body.

Prostaglandins are key players in the body's response to injury or illness. They help create the sensations of pain and inflammation, which are essential for healing but can be problematic when chronic.

Different types of prostaglandins (e.g., PGE2, PGD2, PGF2α, PGI2) have distinct and sometimes opposite effects. For example, while some prostaglandins promote inflammation, others can help resolve it.

In the stomach, prostaglandins protect the lining by stimulating mucus and bicarbonate production, which help neutralize stomach acid and prevent ulcers.

When the body detects an infection, prostaglandins are produced in the brain to raise the body's temperature, causing a fever, which helps fight off the invading pathogens. That is the reason why nonsteroidal anti-inflammatory drugs (NSAIDs) like aspirin, ibuprofen, and naproxen work by inhibiting the enzyme cyclooxygenase (COX), which is crucial for prostaglandin synthesis. Inhibiting prostaglandin production reduces pain, inflammation, and fever.

Prostaglandins help regulate the contraction and relaxation of blood vessel walls, thus controlling blood pressure and the formation of blood clots. They can either promote or inhibit platelet aggregation depending on the type of prostaglandin.

Prostaglandins are involved in causing the uterine contractions that lead to menstrual cramps. High levels of prostaglandins during menstruation can cause more severe cramps and discomfort. Additionally, prostaglandins play a crucial role in childbirth by inducing labor. They help soften the cervix and trigger uterine contractions. Synthetic prostaglandins are sometimes used medically to induce labor.

Prostaglandins can contribute to respiratory conditions like asthma and allergies by causing bronchoconstriction or influencing immune cell activity in the airways.

Some prostaglandins are involved in cancer progression by promoting tumor growth, angiogenesis (formation of new blood vessels), and suppressing the immune response against tumors.

Prostaglandin D2 (PGD2) has been implicated in promoting sleep and regulating the sleep-wake cycle.

How Prostaglandins May Affect Your Skin

As noted earlier, prostaglandins are inflammatory mediators that can lead to skin redness, swelling, and pain. Prostaglandins are also involved in the skin's response to ultraviolet (UV) radiation from the sun, as their overproduction in response to UV exposure can exacerbate skin damage.

They are important in wound healing, as they help regulate the proliferation and migration of skin cells. Yet, excessive production of certain prostaglandins can lead to chronic wounds and poor healing.

Prostaglandins can sensitize nerve endings in the skin, making them more responsive to pain signals. This is why skin trauma, or inflammatory conditions can cause significant discomfort and pain.

Prostaglandins help regulate the skin's moisture barrier. By influencing the production of natural oils and maintaining hydration, they contribute to overall skin health. Disruptions in prostaglandin pathways can lead to dry, flaky skin.

Prostaglandins might play a role in the development and progression of skin cancer. They can promote tumor growth by forming new blood vessels that supply the tumor.

Interesting Facts

Prostaglandins have been found to influence hair growth. For example, certain prostaglandins can promote hair growth, which has led to the development of treatments for conditions like alopecia (hair loss). Originally developed for treating glaucoma and ocular hypertension, latanoprost is a prostaglandin analog that has shown promise in promoting hair growth.

Bimatoprost (brand name Latisse), a synthetic prostaglandin analog, is used to treat inadequate eyelash growth by enhancing eyelash length, thickness, and darkness.

Here is a graphic summary of how prostaglandins can affect common skin diseases.

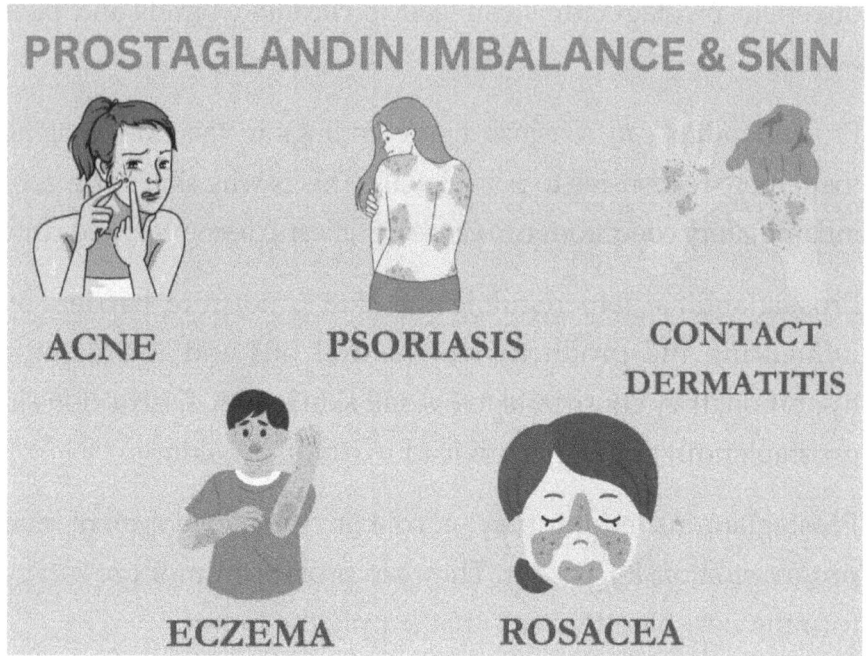

Figure 3.2 Prostaglandin imbalance and skin.

Mediators of Inflammation: Leukotrienes

Similarly to cytokines and prostaglandins, leukotrienes are messengers and orchestrators of complex reactions in our body's inflammatory and immune responses. Like prostaglandins, leukotrienes are lipid compounds. In fact, they are synthesized from arachidonic acid, a fatty acid that is part of the cell membrane. When the body needs to produce leukotrienes, it converts arachidonic acid through the action of the enzyme 5-lipoxygenase. This pathway is crucial for the generation of inflammatory mediators. The protective mechanism of leukotrienes entails attracting white blood cells (leukocytes) to the site of inflammation or infection. This helps coordinate the immune response, ensuring that immune cells are present where they are needed most to fight off harmful substances.

Unfortunately, leukotrienes' claim to fame is mostly related to their severe inflammatory reactions. Here are some of them:

Leukotrienes are major contributors to asthma symptoms. They increase mucus production and cause the airways to narrow (bronchoconstriction), leading to difficulty breathing. They also enhance vascular permeability, leading to symptoms such as wheezing, coughing, and shortness of breath in asthma patients. Because of this, they are a primary target for asthma treatments. By blocking leukotriene pathways, medications, such as montelukast (Singulair) and zafirlukast (Accolate), can help keep the airways open and reduce asthma attacks.

Similarly, leukotrienes play a significant role in anaphylaxis when they are released in large quantities. They contribute to the rapid onset of symptoms by increasing the permeability of blood vessels, causing tissue swelling and bronchoconstriction. This can be life-threatening if not treated immediately.

It is no surprise that leukotrienes are involved in the chronic inflammation seen in conditions like Crohn's disease and ulcerative colitis. By contributing to the inflammatory response in the gut, leukotrienes can exacerbate symptoms such as abdominal pain, diarrhea, and tissue damage. However, this also means that targeting leukotrienes offers a potential therapeutic approach for these conditions, bringing hope for better treatments.

How Leukotrienes May Affect Your Skin

Overactive leukotriene responses can make the skin more sensitive to sunlight, leading to a condition called photodermatitis. In this condition, the skin reacts abnormally to UV exposure, causing rashes, blisters, and severe inflammation.

Here is a graphic representation of the effect of leukotrienes imbalance on common skin conditions.

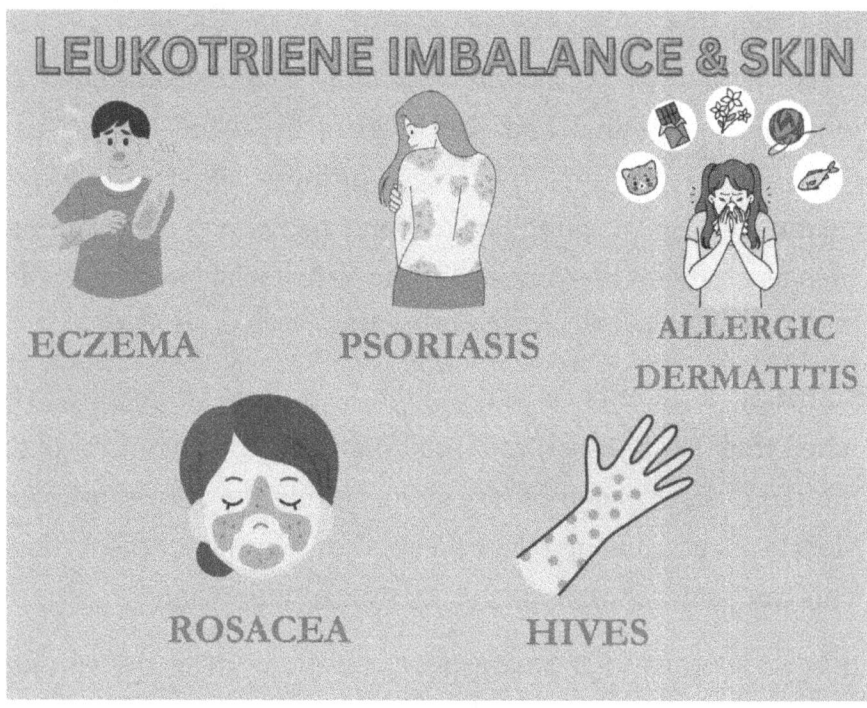

Figure 3.3 Leukotriene imbalance and skin.

CHAPTER 4

Histamine and Food Sensitivities

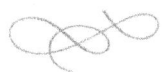

In this chapter, we will examine two often-confused conditions: Mast Cell Activation Syndrome (MCAS) and histamine Intolerance (HIT).

Both involve histamine, a crucial compound in our bodies, but they work in different ways and need different treatments.

All About Histamine

Let's define histamine first.

Have you ever had an allergic reaction, like sneezing around pollen or getting hives from a particular food? That's histamine at work! When your body encounters something it thinks is harmful (like allergens), it releases histamine from special cells called mast cells. Histamine then triggers symptoms like itching, sneezing, or swelling to help your body eliminate the allergen.

Histamine is another chemical messenger involved in the immune, digestive, and central nervous systems. It is produced by the body and is also found in certain foods.

In our digestive system, histamine is involved in producing stomach acid, which is essential for breaking down food. Without enough histamine, your stomach might not produce enough acid, making digestion less efficient.

In your brain, histamine acts as a neurotransmitter, which means it helps send signals between nerve cells. It is essential for regulating sleep-wake cycles, so having the right histamine balance can affect how alert or sleepy you feel.

Sources of Histamine

Your body makes histamine and stores it in several types of cells, such as

- *Mast Cells:* These cells are found in connective tissues throughout the body, particularly in areas prone to injury like the skin, lungs, and gastrointestinal tract. Mast cells play a crucial role in allergic reactions and immune responses.
- *Basophils:* A type of white blood cell found in the bloodstream, basophils also store histamine and are involved in the body's immune response, particularly in allergic reactions.
- *Enterochromaffin-like Cells (ECL Cells):* These cells are located in the stomach lining and release histamine to stimulate the production of gastric acid, aiding in digestion.

- *Neurons:* In the brain, histamine is stored and released by neurons, particularly in the hypothalamus, where it acts as a neurotransmitter to regulate functions such as sleep, appetite, and wakefulness.

Food Sources of Histamine

- *Aged cheeses:* cheddar, gouda, parmesan, Swiss and blue cheese. The bacteria involved in the aging process break down proteins, leading to the formation of histamine.
- *Processed meats:* Processed meats often contain high levels of histamine, particularly those that are cured, smoked, or fermented. Examples include salami, pepperoni, ham, bacon, and sausages.
- *Certain Fish:* Mackerel, tuna, and sardines can be high in histamines, especially if not super fresh.
- *Vegetables:* Tomatoes, eggplants, and spinach are naturally high in histamines.
- *Fermented foods:* Fermented foods are rich in histamine due to the fermentation process, which relies on bacterial action. Common examples are sauerkraut, kimchi, yogurt, kefir, soy sauce, miso, and tempeh. Fermentation enhances the flavor and nutritional profile of these foods but also increases histamine content.
- *Alcoholic beverages,* especially those that are fermented, can contain significant amounts of histamine. Examples include red wine, beer, champagne, whiskey, and vermouth. The fermentation and aging processes involved in producing these beverages contribute to their histamine content. Moreover, alcohol can inhibit the enzyme diamine

oxidase (DAO), which helps break down histamine in the body. By inhibiting the DAO enzyme, alcohol prevents histamine from being metabolized, leading to the accumulation of more histamine.

In addition to skin reactions and respiratory allergies, these foods may cause bloating, nausea, migraines, and sleep disturbance.

How Histamine Works

When histamine is released, it binds to certain receptors in your body. There are four types of histamine receptors, each with different roles:

H1 Receptors

H1 receptors are mainly found on smooth muscle cells, vascular cells, and neurons. They can cause smooth muscle contraction when activated, leading to reactions like bronchoconstriction and intestinal cramping. They also increase vascular permeability, which can result in edema, and stimulate sensory nerve endings, causing itching and pain.

H1 antagonists, commonly known as antihistamines, help alleviate symptoms of allergies and allergic reactions. Common H1 antagonists are diphenhydramine (Benadryl), cetirizine (Zyrtec), and loratadine (Claritin).

H2 Receptors

H2 receptors are primarily located in the stomach lining and are responsible for stimulating gastric acid production. H2 antagonists, or H2 blockers, such as famotidine (Pepcid), are used to decrease stomach acid production. That is the reason they are prescribed to treat GI reflux disease (GERD) and peptic ulcers.

H3 Receptors

H3 receptors are primarily found in the central nervous system (CNS), particularly in areas where neurotransmitters are released and modulated. These important neurotransmitters are dopamine, serotonin, norepinephrine, and acetylcholine.

Research is ongoing to explore H3 receptors as potential targets for neurological and psychiatric disorders.

H4 Receptors

Initially discovered on immune cells such as mast cells, eosinophils, and T cells, H4 receptors are involved in immune responses, including cytokine production. They play a role in inflammation and allergic reactions.

For most people, histamine works smoothly, balancing its various roles without causing problems. However, when histamine levels get too high or your body can't break them down properly, it may result in allergies, digestive issues, or conditions like Histamine Intolerance (HIT).

Understanding histamine helps us appreciate its vital role in keeping our bodies functioning well. Whether fighting off allergens, aiding digestion, or helping us stay alert, histamine is a critical player in our overall health and well-being.

Now let's look in a little more detail at skin issues that are caused by unbalanced histamine production:

How Histamines May Affect Your Skin

- *Rash:* One of the most common signs of too much histamine.
- *Flushing:* Histamines cause the blood vessels in your skin to dilate, leading to that flushed appearance.
- *Itchiness:* Histamines can irritate nerve endings in the skin, leading to itching. This sensation can be bothersome and is a common symptom of allergic reactions. The itchiness caused by histamines can be relentless. Scratching can lead to further irritation and even more histamine release, creating a vicious cycle.
- *Hives (Urticaria):* Histamines are a primary cause of hives. Histamine binds to H1 receptors on the surfaces of blood vessels, leading to the dilation (widening) and increased permeability of these vessels. The increased permeability allows fluid from the cells to leak into the surrounding tissues.
- *Angioedema:* In some cases, histamines can cause angioedema, a deeper swelling affecting areas like the eyelids, lips, and throat. This condition can be more severe than hives and requires prompt medical attention.

Mast Cell Activation Syndrome (MCAS)

Mast cells are everywhere in your body, especially in organs like your skin, lungs, and digestive system. They have granules packed with histamine and other chemicals released in response to allergens, infections, or injuries. Typically, this release is controlled, but in MCAS, it's not.

Mast Cell Activation Syndrome happens when mast cells release large quantities of biochemical substances, such as histamine, prostaglandins, cytokines, leukotrienes, and proteases.

Proteases are like tiny scissors in your body, constantly cutting proteins into smaller pieces. Imagine you have a big, tangled ball of yarn (proteins) that needs to be cut into shorter, manageable strands. Proteases do this job, ensuring proteins are in the right shape and size to be used effectively by your body.

There are different types of proteases, each with a specific job and target. For example, digestive proteases, such as pepsin in the stomach and trypsin in the intestines, help digest the proteins in your food.

Proteases help your immune system by breaking down harmful proteins from bacteria and viruses. This enables your body to fight off infections more effectively.

Inside your cells, proteases help get rid of damaged or unnecessary proteins, keeping everything running smoothly.

In the blood, proteases help with blood clotting.

Fun Fact

Did you know that proteases are also used outside the body? They are added to laundry detergents to help break down protein stains on your clothes, like blood or food. They're also used in the food industry to tenderize meat and make it easier to chew.

Symptoms of MCAS

- ❖ *Skin:* Hives, flushing, and swelling (angioedema).
- ❖ *Digestive System:* Nausea, vomiting, diarrhea, and abdominal pain.
- ❖ *Respiratory System:* Wheezing, shortness of breath, and nasal congestion.
- ❖ *Heart and Blood Vessels:* Low blood pressure, fast heart rate, and shock
- ❖ *Nervous System:* Headaches, difficulty concentrating, and lightheadedness.

Diagnosis of MCAS

Due to its wide range of symptoms, MCAS may be hard to diagnose. Here are the components of evaluation to help with that:

- ❖ *Clinical Evaluation*: Detailed symptom history and physical exam.
- ❖ *Laboratory Tests*: Checking levels of tryptase, histamine, prostaglandins, and leukotrienes in the blood.
- ❖ *Response to Treatment*: Monitoring if symptoms improve with treatments like antihistamines and leukotriene inhibitors.

Treating MCAS

Managing MCAS means controlling symptoms and preventing mast cells from releasing chemicals. It includes:

- ❖ *Medications:* Antihistamines, mast cell stabilizers, leukotriene inhibitors, and sometimes corticosteroids.

- *Low-Histamine Diet:* Avoid high-histamine foods, as well as foods like strawberries and citrus fruits, which are not high in histamine but can trigger histamine release.

  The list includes foods with high tyramine content, as tyramines can also cause histamine release. Tyramine is an amino acid that accumulates in various aged, fermented, cured, and processed foods due to protein breakdown. These foods, which include aged cheeses, cured meats, and fermented products, tend to have higher tyramine levels due to the aging and fermentation processes.

  Food Additives, such as preservatives (such as sulfites and benzoates), artificial colors, and flavor enhancers (such as monosodium glutamate or MSG), should be avoided.

  Leftover foods can also increase in histamine content the longer they are stored.

Medications to Avoid:

- **NSAIDs**: Non-steroidal anti-inflammatory drugs like ibuprofen and aspirin
- **Opioids**: Medications like morphine and codeine.
- **Certain Antibiotics**: Such as quinolones and vancomycin.
- **Contrast Dyes**: Both oral and intravenous contract dye, like the one used in CAT scans, should be avoided.

Environmental Factors:

- **Temperature Extremes**: Both hot and cold temperatures can trigger symptoms.
- **Strong Odors**: Perfumes, scented products, and chemical fumes.

- **Pollens and Molds**: Common allergens can trigger mast cell activation.
- **Insect Stings/Bites**: Venoms can cause significant mast cell degranulation.

Stress

- **Physical Stress**: Intense exercise or physical exertion.
- **Emotional Stress**: Anxiety, depression, or significant life changes can exacerbate symptoms.

Histamine Intolerance (HIT)

Histamine Intolerance (HIT) occurs when there's an excess of histamine in the body that cannot be broken down quickly enough. Usually, histamine is metabolized by specific enzymes:

- *Diamine Oxidase (DAO)* primarily breaks down histamine in the gut. We have discussed earlier how alcohol blocks this enzyme.
- *Histamine-N-Methyltransferase (HNMT)* breaks down histamine in various tissues, such as the liver, kidney, brain, and lung.

When these enzymes do not function effectively, histamine accumulates in the body, leading to various symptoms.

Symptoms of HIT

HIT symptoms are similar to allergic reactions and affect most body systems:

- *Skin:* Flushing, hives, and rash.
- *Digestive System:* Bloating, diarrhea, and stomach cramps.

- *Respiratory System:* Nasal congestion, sneezing, and asthma-like symptoms.
- *Heart and Blood Vessels:* Headaches, palpitations, and low or high blood pressure.
- *Nervous System:* Fatigue, dizziness, and irritability.

Diagnosis of HIT

Clinical components of HIT include:

- *Clinical symptom history:* Keeping a food diary and correlating symptoms with food intake.
- *Enzyme Activity Test:* Measuring DAO activity in the blood.
- *Elimination Diet:* Removing high-histamine foods from the diet and tracking if symptoms improve.

Treating HIT

Managing HIT focuses on reducing histamine intake and helping the body break it down. These interventions include:

- *Low-Histamine Diet:* Avoid foods high in histamine and eat fresh, unprocessed foods.
- *Supplements:* Take DAO supplements and micronutrients that support DAO activity, such as vitamin B6, vitamin C, copper, zinc, magnesium, and calcium.
- *Medications:* Take antihistamines and avoid substances that inhibit DAO.
- *Lifestyle:* Manage stress and stay well-hydrated.

Key Differences Between MCAS and HIT

Mechanism of Action

- ❖ *MCAS*: Involves the uncontrolled release of chemicals from mast cells, affecting many systems.
- ❖ *HIT*: Happens when there is too much histamine, and the body can't break it down fast enough.

Symptoms

- ❖ *MCAS*: Causes a wide range of severe symptoms that come and go.
- ❖ *HIT*: Symptoms are mainly related to histamine in the diet and often mimic allergies.

Diagnosis

- ❖ *MCAS*: Identified by high levels of mast cell chemicals and response to treatment.
- ❖ *HIT*: Diagnosed by tracking symptoms with food intake, measuring DAO activity, and trying a low-histamine diet.

Treatment

- ❖ *MCAS*: Needs a mix of antihistamines, mast cell stabilizers, leukotriene inhibitors, and dietary changes.
- ❖ *HIT*: Managed with dietary restrictions, DAO supplements, and antihistamines.

To sum up, while both conditions involve issues with histamine, MCAS is a more concerning disease due to its potential severity, systemic impact, and the complexity of its management. It is essential for individuals with either condition to work closely with healthcare providers to develop an appropriate management plan.

CHAPTER 5

Gut-Skin Axis and Food Sensitivities

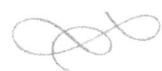

Let's start our discussion by defining gut permeability, gut microbiome, and gut inflammation.

These terms have been making waves lately, especially in the world of functional and integrative medicine, where both concepts are closely intertwined.

Dysfunctional gut is at the core of many skin and non-skin diseases, so we will go into some interesting details in this chapter.

Definitions: Leaky Gut, Gut Microbiome, and Gut Inflammation

Gut Permeability

To better understand gut permeability, it's useful to first learn about the structure and function of your gut. Your gastrointestinal (GI) tract is a sophisticated system built to digest and absorb nutrients. Additionally, it acts as a vital barrier, protecting your body's internal environment from external elements.

The gut lining, or intestinal epithelium, comprises a single layer of cells known as enterocytes. These cells are held together by tight junctions, which regulate what can pass through the gut lining. This is important because it allows nutrients into your bloodstream while keeping harmful substances like toxins and pathogens out.

A leaky gut occurs when tight junctions in the gut lining become loosened or disrupted. When this barrier is compromised, larger molecules like undigested food particles, toxins, and microbes can pass through and enter the bloodstream. This can trigger immune responses and cause inflammation, both in the gut and throughout the body.

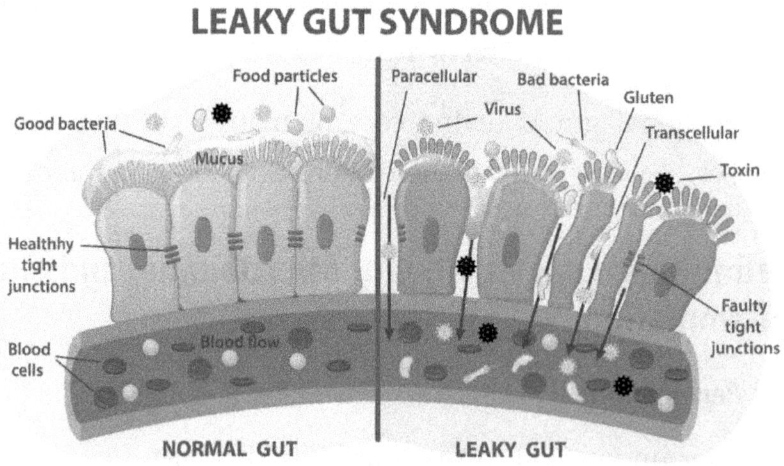

Figure 5.1 Leaky gut

Gut Microbiome

The gut microbiome is essentially a complex community of trillions of microorganisms residing in your digestive tract.

Here are the types of microorganisms that constitute the human gut microbiome:

- *Bacteria*: These are the most abundant and well-known members of the gut microbiome. They help with digestion, produce essential nutrients, and protect against harmful invaders. Some of the most common beneficial bacteria are *Lactobacillus* and *Bifidobacterium*.
- **Viruses:** While some viruses can cause illnesses, many are harmless or even beneficial. The most common types found in the gut are bacteriophages, which infect bacteria and help control their populations.
- *Fungi*: Fungi, like yeasts, are also part of the gut microbiome. They assist in digestion and nutrient absorption in small amounts, but their overgrowth can lead to problems like infections.
- *Archaea*: These single-celled organisms resemble bacteria but have different genetic structures. They help break down complex sugars and produce methane, which is involved in digestion.
- *Protozoa*: These single-celled eukaryotes help manage the population of bacteria and other microorganisms in the gut. While some protozoa can cause diseases, many live peacefully within the gut environment.

Why is Gut Microbiome Important?

The gut microbiome is essential for several reasons:

- ❖ *Digestion:* The gut microbiome aids digestion by breaking down complex carbohydrates, proteins, and fibers that the human body cannot digest on its own, producing beneficial short-chain fatty acids and essential vitamins. It also enhances nutrient absorption, supports gut barrier integrity, and helps detoxify harmful substances.
- ❖ *Nutrient Production:* Some gut bacteria produce essential vitamins like B12 and K, which are crucial for various bodily functions.
- ❖ *Immune System Support:* The gut microbiome is essential for the development and function of the immune system, helping to protect against harmful pathogens.
- ❖ *Mental Health:* The gut-brain communication is called the gut-brain axis. Mood disorders and our cognitive function are impacted by this connection.

Leaky gut and microbiome dysbalance usually have similar etiologies, such as poor diet, infections, toxins, etc.

Unsurprisingly, microbiome dysbalance is often the primary cause of leaky gut. Fixing the gut microbiome may improve or even reverse the condition.

Gut Inflammation

Chronic inflammation in the gut can weaken the tight junctions that help preserve the integrity of the intestinal mucosa. This inflammation can be instigated by many triggers, including, but not limited to, infections, food sensitivities, and autoimmune conditions. When these threats are detected, the immune system responds by producing inflammatory substances, such as the ones we discussed previously: cytokines, prostaglandins, and leukotrienes. Let us not forget that 70% of the immune system resides in our gut. While intended to combat the threats, these substances can also disrupt the gut barrier, resulting in a leaky gut. This compromise in barrier allows toxic and harmful substances to enter the bloodstream, potentially causing further inflammation and contributing to various health issues.

Now, let's move on to the causes of leaky gut and start with the most important one.

Causes of Leaky Gut: Poor Diet

In Western society, there are many diet and lifestyle-related causes of leaky gut, such as diets rich in sugar and processed foods, infections, exposure to toxins (plastic, environmental), medications, stress, autoimmune conditions, metabolic conditions (diabetes, and metabolic syndrome), inflammatory bowel disease (both cause and result of a leaky gut), and malnutrition in terms of the availability of essential nutrients.

Of all these factors, poor diet contributes the most to leaky gut and our general health. Unfortunately, it cannot be undone by exercise and addition of supplements. They help but cannot reverse the harm being done by daily ingestion of harmful substances. Yes, the Western diet qualifies as a diet full of harmful and toxic for our body substances. The effects of this diet range from immediate ones, such as bloating and headache, to lifelong ones, such as diabetes and heart disease.

Components of Poor Diet or Foods to Avoid:

- ❖ *Processed Foods*: Essential components of processed foods are additives, preservatives, and low-quality ingredients that can damage the gut lining, leading to inflammation and weakening the tight junctions that help maintain gut integrity.
- ❖ *Fast Food:* Burgers, fries, and other restaurant-fried foods are typically loaded with unhealthy fats, refined carbohydrates, and artificial additives. These components can promote inflammation and disrupt the gut microbiome.
- ❖ *Snack Foods*: Chips, crackers, and other packaged snacks often contain trans fats, high levels of sodium, and artificial flavors. Trans fats cause inflammation and can negatively affect gut barrier function.
- ❖ *Frozen Meals:* Many frozen dinners are high in preservatives, sodium, and unhealthy fats, all of which can contribute to a leaky gut. These meals often lack fiber and essential nutrients that support gut health, further exacerbating gut issues.
- ❖ *Sugar:* High sugar intake is particularly damaging to the gut. Sugars feed harmful bacteria and yeast, leading to gut dysbiosis. Familiar sources of excessive sugar include:

    <u>Sugary Beverages:</u> Sodas, energy drinks, and sweetened coffee or tea are major sources of added sugars. These beverages can spike blood sugar levels, creating a favorable environment for harmful bacteria and yeast in the gut.

    <u>Sweets and Desserts:</u> Cakes, cookies, candies, and ice cream contribute significantly to high sugar consump-

tion. These foods feed harmful microbes and promote inflammation, which can damage the gut.

Hidden Sugars: Many packaged foods, including seemingly healthy options like granola bars and yogurt, can contain high levels of added sugars. The hidden sugars in these products can disrupt the gut microbiome balance, leading to increased gut permeability.

Unhealthy Fats:

Diets high in unhealthy fats, particularly trans fats and saturated fats, can also negatively affect gut health. Examples include:

Fried Foods: Deep-fried items like doughnuts, fried chicken, and fries are high in trans fats. Trans fats cause inflammation and have been linked to an increased incidence of chronic diseases, which can be exacerbated by poor gut health.

Baked Goods: Many store-bought baked goods, such as pastries, cookies, and cakes, contain trans fats and saturated fats.

Processed Meats: Hot dogs, sausages, and other processed meats are known for high saturated fats and additives.

We will discuss in detail the foods that support and heal gut and diversify microbiome in *Chapter 21. Clear Skin Diet.*

Let's move on to medications that can cause gut problems.

Causes of Leaky Gut: Nonsteroidal Anti-Inflammatory Drugs (NSAIDs)

NSAIDs are used to alleviate pain, decrease inflammation, and reduce fevers. Common NSAIDs include ibuprofen (Advil, Motrin), aspirin (Bayer, Bufferin), and naproxen (Aleve).

While effective, NSAIDs can cause direct damage to the gut lining. This damage occurs because NSAIDs inhibit the production of prostaglandins, which, as we learned earlier, are compounds that help maintain the protective mucus lining of the gut. Without sufficient prostaglandins, the mucus layer thins out, making the gut lining more susceptible to damage from stomach acids and digestive enzymes. This reduces mucus and bicarbonate (alkaline) secretion, making the stomach lining more vulnerable to injury from stomach acid and digestive enzymes.

Additionally, NSAID-induced damage to the gut lining can weaken tight junctions, allowing harmful substances to pass into the bloodstream by decreasing gut permeability.

Due to their effects on the gut, usage of NSAIDs can lead to the following medical conditions:

NSAID-induced Gastritis

The symptoms of gastritis caused by NSAIDs can vary in severity, from mild and occasional to bothersome and frequent. They may include abdominal pain, often experienced as a burning or gnawing sensation in the upper abdomen. This pain may improve or worsen with eating. Nausea and vomiting are also common symptoms. In some cases, vomiting may include blood or material that looks like coffee grounds, indicating bleeding in the stomach. Other symptoms include bloating, belching, a loss of appetite, indigestion, and black or tarry stools, which signify gastrointestinal bleeding.

NSAID- induced Peptic Ulcers

Peptic ulcers are open sores or crater-like ulcerations that form within the lining of the stomach or upper small intestine. Similarly to gastritis, peptic ulcers form when stomach acid and digestive enzymes erode the protective mucus of the stomach or small intestine.

The symptoms of peptic ulcers are remarkably similar to those of gastritis, and the best way to diagnose either condition is with an upper endoscopy or esophagogastroduodenoscopy (EGD). During this procedure, a camera is threaded through the mouth into the stomach and upper small intestine. This allows the visualization of gastritis and/or ulcers directly, and biopsies are taken to establish and confirm the diagnosis.

Laboratory tests may also be conducted to check for anemia, which can result from chronic bleeding, and to diagnose the presence of Helicobacter pylori bacteria that can also cause ulcers and may coexist with NSAID-induced ulcers. H.pylori has been known to exacerbate both gastritis and peptic ulcers, and it has been linked to the development of stomach cancer.

The presence of H.pylori may start a destructive domino effect by lowering the gastric acid in the stomach and creating a sustainable environment for the overgrowth of bacteria that would have stayed dormant otherwise. (In some cases, H.pylori can increase the secretion of gastric acid.) This may trigger various diseases, from SIBO (Small Intestine Bacterial Overgrowth) to skin conditions, such as eczema, and neurological diseases, such as Alzheimer's dementia.

The essential step in the treatment of NSAID-induced gastritis and peptic ulcers is discontinuing NSAIDs!

If discontinuation is not possible, switching to a different pain reliever, such as acetaminophen (Tylenol), which does not have the same gastrointestinal side effects, may be recommended. However, acetaminophen may not address the pain in the same way as NSAIDs, and this presents a challenge for a clinician in addressing the patient's pain for which the NSAIDs were prescribed in the first place. Additionally, acetaminophen is not the best choice for somebody with liver problems, as it is metabolized in the liver.

Always consult your healthcare provider before making any changes in your medication regimen.

Causes of Leaky Gut: Antibiotics

Antibiotics are life-saving drugs that fight off bacterial infections. They work by killing bacteria or preventing them from multiplying. While this is great for getting rid of harmful bacteria causing infections, antibiotics don't discriminate between the bad bacteria and the good ones.

When you take antibiotics, especially broad-spectrum ones, they wipe out beneficial bacteria. As you recall, beneficial bacteria in your gut help maintain the integrity of the gut lining.

They produce substances that nourish the cells of the gut lining and keep the tight junctions intact. When antibiotics reduce the population of these good bacteria, it can weaken the gut barrier, making it more permeable.

With good bacteria out of the way, harmful bacteria and yeast can overgrow (bacterial overgrowth). This dysbiosis can lead to inflammation and damage to the gut lining. Inflammatory substances produced by these harmful bacteria can further loosen the tight junctions, contributing to a leaky gut.

In addition to triggering harmful bacteria to activate an inflammatory cascade, antibiotics can sometimes cause direct inflammation in the gut. This inflammation can damage the cells of the gut lining and the tight junctions, increasing gut permeability and thus allowing harmful substances and toxins to be absorbed into your bloodstream.

Strategies to Protect Your Gut While Taking Antibiotics

- ❖ *Probiotics and Prebiotics:* It is important to take probiotics and prebiotics (fiber for beneficial bacteria in probiotics) while on antibiotics (see *Chapter 21. Clear Skin Diet* for more details on natural and supplemental forms of both).
- ❖ *Diet:* See *Chapter 21. Clear Skin Diet*
- ❖ *Drink Water*, as good hydration, is essential for the mucosal lining of the intestines and helps maintain the integrity of the gut barrier.

Avoid Unnecessary Antibiotics:

Only use antibiotics when absolutely necessary and as prescribed by your healthcare provider. Overusing and misusing antibiotics can raise the risk of antibiotic resistance and harm your gut health.

Always consult your healthcare provider before making any changes in your medication regimen.

Causes of Leaky Gut: Proton Pump Inhibitors (PPIs)

The primary role of PPIs is to reduce stomach acid production. They are frequently prescribed for conditions such as gastroesophageal reflux disease (GERD), stomach ulcers, and other acid-related disorders. Common PPIs include omeprazole (Prilosec), esomeprazole (Nexium), lansoprazole (Prevacid), and pantoprazole (Protonix).

While PPIs are effective in managing acid-related conditions, there is growing concern about their long-term use and potential side effects, including their impact on gut health and the possible development of leaky gut syndrome.

Stomach acid plays a vital role in digestion by breaking down food and eliminating harmful bacteria and pathogens. By significantly reducing stomach acid, PPIs can disrupt normal digestive processes and alter the gut environment. Altering the gut microbiome can lead to SIBO, an overgrowth of bacteria in the stomach and small intestine. It can also contribute to gut inflammation and increased intestinal permeability.

Another essential role of stomach acid is that it is necessary for the absorption of certain nutrients, such as magnesium, calcium, and vitamin B12. Long-term use of PPIs can lead to deficiencies in these nutrients, compromising gut health and overall well-being.

Strategies to Mitigate the Impact of PPIs on Gut Health

- *Probiotics:* Eating probiotic-rich foods and/or taking a probiotic supplement can help balance gut bacteria and reduce the risk of SIBO. However, if there is a high suspicion for SIBO, then probiotics may aggravate it, so please consult your healthcare provider before starting them. Sometimes, a slower introduction of the lower dosages is implemented.
- *Nutrient Supplementation:* Supplementing with magnesium, calcium, and vitamin B12 can help prevent deficiencies associated with long-term PPI use.
- *Diet*: See *Chapter 21. Clear Skin Diet*
- *Medical Supervision:* Regular assessment by your clinician should determine the necessity of ongoing PPI therapy and evaluate potential side effects.

Discussing alternative treatments for acid-related conditions, such as H2 blockers or lifestyle changes (e.g., dietary modifications, weight loss, and avoiding trigger foods), can also be beneficial.

Limiting the use of PPIs to the shortest duration necessary can reduce the risk of developing complications associated with long-term use. Sometimes it may not be feasible.

While PPIs are effective in managing acid-related disorders, their long-term use can potentially contribute to gut health issues, including increased gut permeability or leaky gut.

As always, please consult with your clinician before changing your medication regimen.

Causes of Leaky Gut: Chronic Stress

One of the most important questions a clinician should ask a patient with a new or persistent skin issue is whether a specific stressful situation precipitated it in the first place. In some cases, there is a clear correlation between a stressful event and the onset of a new skin problem. Alternatively, patients can report the constant daily stress they have lived with for a long time. In that case, we are dealing with cumulative stress, the detrimental effects of which may be equally challenging to remedy for both the patient and the clinician.

Cortisol is the hormone our body produces when we are stressed. While cortisol is essential for managing short-term stress, prolonged stress and constant high levels of cortisol can have profoundly detrimental effects on our health in general, including the gut.

Cortisol can make the tight junctions in the gut lining more permeable, induce gut inflammation, and lead to gut dysbiosis.

Your gut and brain are intricately connected through the gut-brain axis, a sophisticated communication network that links mood and thought centers with intestinal functions. Stress can alter this communication, affecting gut health in several ways.

Cortisol can influence this communication, potentially leading to gastrointestinal discomfort, nausea, and changes in bowel habits.

Symptoms of a "nervous stomach" due to cortisol include nausea, butterflies in the stomach (related to a change in blood flow and gut motility in response to stress), stomach cramps and pain, and diarrhea or constipation due to altered motility. These symptoms may seem familiar to some because they sound remarkably similar to IBS.

Indeed, chronic stress through cortisol fluctuations may lead to IBS.

Cortisol can increase the production of stomach acid, which may lead to symptoms such as heartburn, indigestion, and acid reflux. That is why chronic stress has been linked to the development of peptic ulcers and gastritis.

Strategies to Mitigate the Effects of Cortisol on the Gut

- ❖ ***Stress Management Techniques***: Practices such as mindfulness, meditation, yoga, and deep breathing exercises can help reduce cortisol levels and alleviate symptoms of a nervous stomach.
- ❖ ***Diet:*** See *Chapter 21. Clear Skin Diet*
- ❖ ***Regular Exercise***: Physical activity can help regulate the stress response and reduce cortisol levels.
- ❖ ***Adequate Sleep***: Ensuring adequate sleep can help regulate cortisol levels and improve overall stress resilience.

- *Hydration:* Staying well-hydrated supports overall digestive health and can help mitigate some gastrointestinal symptoms associated with stress.

We will discuss cortisol in more detail in *Chapter 6. Hormones and Food Sensitivities*.

Causes of Leaky Gut: Infections

Infections can significantly impact the gut lining and contribute to a leaky gut. In addition to causing inflammation and inducing gut dysbiosis, they can cause direct damage to the gut lining.

Here are some examples:

- *Bacterial Infections:* Certain harmful bacteria, like *Salmonella, E. coli,* and *Clostridium difficile,* can produce toxins that damage the gut lining. These toxins disrupt the tight junctions between cells, making the gut barrier more permeable.
- *Viral Infections:* Viruses like norovirus or rotavirus can infect the gut lining cells, causing inflammation and damage that lead to increased permeability.
- *Parasitic Infections:* Parasites such as Giardia can attach to the gut lining, cause physical damage, and trigger inflammatory responses that weaken the gut barrier.
- *Fungal infections*, such as Candida, can contribute to a leaky gut.

Leaky Gut and Various Medical Conditions

In the world of functional medicine, a healthy gut is considered the foundation of health. In fact, in approach to many diseases, the gut assessment is the first step in evaluating the patient's whole being. Not only does it help to diagnose a leaky gut, but it also helps to point the functional medicine provider in the right direction in terms of connecting the lines between the leaky gut and other medical conditions. In this chapter, we will briefly discuss conditions linked to a leaky gut. Still, this list and the chapter could have been much longer if our goal were to include all gut-related diseases. Let's look at some of them.

Gastrointestinal Diseases

Irritable Bowel Syndrome (IBS)

For a long time, IBS was not considered a real condition and was labeled as a "nervous stomach." There is no need to prove that it is real now, but this label of "nervous stomach" has some truth to it.

Due to the gut-brain connection, psychological factors such as stress and anxiety can affect gut motility, secretion, and sensitivity, exacerbating IBS symptoms.

Meanwhile, other components of the leaky gut are often present. Reduced diversity of gut bacteria has been observed in IBS patients, creating gut microbiome dysbalance. This dysbiosis can lead to increased gas production, altered gut motility, and inflammation, all of which contribute to IBS symptoms.

Some studies suggest that individuals with IBS may have increased intestinal permeability, allowing antigens (substances that the body sees as foreign to it) and toxins to cross the gut barrier and trigger immune responses and inflammation. The leakage of gut contents into the bloodstream can lead to low-grade inflammation and immune activation, contributing to IBS symptoms.

IBS is characterized by abnormal gut motility, leading to symptoms such as diarrhea, constipation, or a mix of both. This can result from disruptions in the normal rhythmic contractions of the gut muscles. Individuals with IBS often experience heightened sensitivity to pain and discomfort in the gut, known as visceral hypersensitivity. This can make normal gut movements and gas more painful.

While IBS is not primarily an inflammatory condition like Inflammatory Bowel Disease (IBD) (see next), some patients exhibit low-grade inflammation in the gut, which can contribute to symptoms.

Inflammatory Bowel Disease (IBD)

Both Crohn's disease and ulcerative colitis are heavily connected to a leaky gut. Several components of gut issues play a role in IBD, such as compromise of tight junctions, gut inflammation, gut dysbiosis, and the trigger of immune response by the leakage of antigens from the gut into the bloodstream. These are serious diseases that often lead to bleeding, bowel obstructions, and surgeries. Ulcerative colitis may often be a precursor to colon cancer.

Autoimmune Diseases

Rheumatoid Arthritis (RA)

Rheumatoid arthritis is a chronic autoimmune disorder characterized by inflammation of the joints. It occurs when the immune system mistakenly attacks the synovium—the lining of the membranes surrounding the joints—causing pain, swelling, stiffness, and, eventually, joint damage. RA can also affect other organs and systems in the body, leading to fatigue, fever, and systemic inflammation. The exact cause of RA is unknown, but genetic, environmental, and hormonal factors are thought to contribute. One of the causes that has been linked to RA is gut dysbiosis and leaky gut. In fact, specific bacteria, such as *Prevotella copri*, have been associated with the development of RA.

Lupus

Lupus is a whole-body autoimmune disease that can affect the skin, joints, kidneys, and other organs.

Research has found increased intestinal permeability in lupus patients compared to healthy controls. This increased permeability correlates with higher levels of inflammatory markers and disease activity in lupus.

Additionally, individuals with a genetic predisposition to lupus may be more susceptible to the effects of a leaky gut, leading to a heightened immune response.

Multiple Sclerosis (MS)

Multiple sclerosis is a long-term disease where the immune system mistakenly attacks the nerves in the brain and spinal cord, causing various physical and mental problems. Gut dysbiosis is often observed in individuals with MS. Studies have found higher levels of intestinal permeability and altered gut microbiota in MS patients compared to healthy controls. These changes correlate with disease activity and severity.

Mental Health

Depression

There are several mechanisms linking depression and gut issues, such as increased gut permeability (leaky gut) and leakage of antigens into the bloodstream, resulting in an immune response. Inflammation associated with leaky gut increases the production of pro-inflammatory cytokines such as interleukin-6 (IL-6) and tumor necrosis factor-alpha (TNF-α). These cytokines can cross the blood-brain barrier and cause inflammation in the brain, affecting brain signaling pathways involved in mood regulation.

Chronic inflammation and immune activation can dysregulate the hypothalamic-pituitary-adrenal (HPA) axis, leading to altered cortisol levels and contributing to depressive symptoms.

A significant portion of the body's serotonin, a key neurotransmitter in mood regulation, is produced in the gut. Leaky gut and dysbiosis can affect serotonin production and availability, influencing depression. In the same vein, inflammation can alter the metabolism of tryptophan, an amino acid precursor to serotonin, leading to reduced serotonin levels and increased production of metabolites that may contribute to depression.

Anxiety

The mechanism of gut influence on anxiety is similar to the one of depression, but there are a few differences.

Anxiety can be triggered by more acute inflammatory responses and immediate stress signaling, while depression is more strongly linked to chronic inflammation and long-term alterations in neurotransmitter levels.

Anxiety is more linked to imbalances in gamma-aminobutyric acid (GABA), and glutamate, as well as serotonin. The gut microbiota influences the production of GABA, an inhibitory neurotransmitter. Gut dysbiosis can reduce GABA levels, which is associated with increased anxiety.

Both conditions involve problems with the HPA axis, ultimately leading to cortisol production, but in different ways. Anxiety is more often linked to constant overactivity of the HPA axis, while depression can cause the HPA axis to sometimes be overactive and other times be underactive.

Brain Fog

A leaky gut has been associated with difficulty concentrating and memory issues. Some patterns of gut issues are noted in individuals suffering from it, such as increased permeability, leakage of antigens into the bloodstream, cytokine production, and gut dysbiosis, leading to altered serotonin and tryptophan production. It should be added that a leaky gut may lead to or exacerbate nutritional deficiencies, which can also contribute to brain fog.

Latest Research

Leaky Gut and Alzheimer's Disease

Recent studies have shown that inflammation associated with leaky gut and gut dysbiosis can cross the blood-brain barrier and promote neuroinflammation, a key factor in Alzheimer's Disease (AD) progression. Some gut bacteria produce amyloid-like particles, which may seed the formation of amyloid plaques in the brain, a hallmark of AD. Specific changes in the gut microbiome can serve as early biomarkers for AD, potentially allowing for earlier diagnosis and intervention.

Leaky Gut and Parkinson's Disease

It has been observed that many Parkinson's Disease (PD) patients experience gastrointestinal issues such as constipation years before motor symptoms appear. The misfolded protein alpha-synuclein, a hallmark of PD, is found in the gut and is hypothesized to spread from the gut to the brain via the vagus nerve. Additionally, dysbiosis, or an imbalance in gut bacteria, is commonly observed in PD patients, potentially contributing to systemic inflammation and affecting the gut-brain axis. Chronic inflammation in the gut can lead to neuroinflammation, playing a role in the neurodegenerative processes of PD. Understanding the gut-brain axis opens new therapeutic avenues, including probiotics, prebiotics, and dietary interventions aimed at restoring a healthy gut microbiome to potentially slow or alter the progression of PD.

Now, we are getting closer to looking into a connection between leaky gut and food sensitivities.

Leaky Gut and Food Sensitivities: Bidirectional Relationship

We have discussed that in a healthy gut, the intestinal lining acts as a barrier, tightly regulating what passes into the bloodstream. In a leaky gut, the tight junctions between intestinal cells become compromised, allowing larger molecules and undigested food particles to pass through. When undigested food particles leak into the bloodstream, the immune system identifies them as foreign invaders (antigens).

The immune system responds by producing antibodies against these food particles. Over time, this can lead to the development of food sensitivities as the body mounts an immune response every time the specific food is consumed. The presence of foreign particles in the bloodstream triggers an inflammatory response. Chronic inflammation can further damage the intestinal lining, perpetuating the cycle of a leaky gut. This inflammation can have systemic effects, contributing to various symptoms associated with food sensitivities, such as gastrointestinal discomfort, skin reactions, and fatigue. Dysbiosis, which is often associated with a leaky gut, can exacerbate inflammation and immune system dysregulation, further promoting food sensitivities.

How Food Sensitivities May Aggravate Leaky Gut

Food sensitivities can aggravate leaky gut through similar mechanisms, such as activating the immune system, creating or escalating inflammation, and producing cytokines.

Additionally, foods can directly attack the epithelial lining of the gut by releasing certain substances, such as histamine. Some food sensitivities can lead to bacterial overgrowth, thus contributing to gut dysbiosis.

Sometimes, molecular mimicry occurs when certain food particles resemble the body's own tissues, leading to autoimmune reactions. The immune system may attack both the food particles and similar-looking body tissues, causing further damage and symptoms.

Research has shown that individuals with food sensitivities often have higher levels of inflammatory markers and increased intestinal permeability.

In short, the relationship between leaky gut and food sensitivities is bidirectional, with each contributing to the other. That is why healing our gut can make a big difference in the persistence and degree of food sensitivities.

> *Interesting Fact*
>
> **The Impact of C-Section on Gut Microbiota**
>
> Babies born via C-section often experience different initial colonization of gut bacteria compared to those born vaginally. This difference can affect their gut health in several ways. C-section births bypass the natural exposure to the mother's

vaginal and intestinal microbiota. Instead, these babies are initially colonized by bacteria from the hospital environment and the skin, which can lead to a less diverse and less beneficial gut microbiota. The lack of early exposure to beneficial bacteria can increase the risk of gut dysbiosis, making these infants more susceptible to gut permeability issues and subsequent food sensitivities or allergies. Additionally, the babies born via C-section might have delayed or altered immune system development, increasing their susceptibility to allergies and autoimmune conditions.

Let's look at how a leaky gut may affect our skin.

Acne And Leaky Gut

A leaky gut can contribute to acne through several interconnected mechanisms that we have already reviewed, such as:

- ❖ *Increased Intestinal Permeability* allows bacteria, toxins, and undigested food particles to enter the bloodstream and trigger an immune response, resulting in skin inflammation, manifesting as pimples, redness, and skin irritation.
- ❖ *Systemic Inflammation* accompanied by the production of pro-inflammatory cytokines such as IL-6, TNF-α, and IL-1β. These cytokines can circulate throughout the body, contributing to inflammation in the skin by stimulating the skin's sebaceous (oil) glands and hair follicles.
- ❖ *Hormonal Imbalance* due to chronic inflammation from the gut may lead to increasing levels of androgens

(testosterone and DHT), which can stimulate sebaceous glands and lead to increased sebum production.
- ❖ *Gut Dysbiosis*, as part of which harmful bacteria in a dysbiotic gut can produce endotoxins, such as lipopolysaccharides (LPS), which can enter the bloodstream due to a leaky gut. These endotoxins can trigger inflammatory responses in the skin, contributing to acne.

Eczema and Psoriasis and Leaky Gut

While leaky gut influences both eczema and psoriasis through mechanisms involving increased intestinal permeability, systemic inflammation, and dysbiosis, the specific immune pathways and clinical manifestations differ.

Immune Response:

Eczema: The immune response to eczema is often characterized by an overproduction of IgG and IgE antibodies, which leads to hypersensitivity reactions and skin inflammation.

Psoriasis: Psoriasis involves an autoimmune response in which special immune cells, called T-cells, attack healthy skin cells, leading to rapid skin cell turnover and plaque formation. The Th17 pathway, which produces cytokines like IL-17, plays a significant role in psoriasis. This mechanism is different from the production of immunoglobulins.

Clinical Manifestations:

Eczema: Typically presents with itchy, inflamed, and often oozing skin lesions. It is often associated with a history of allergies or asthma.

Psoriasis: Characterized by thick, red, scaly patches on the skin, often on the elbows, knees, and scalp. It is less commonly associated with other allergic conditions.

Often, patients use eczema and psoriasis interchangeably. However, they are two entities with different action mechanisms and clinical manifestations. Addressing gut health may benefit both conditions, though the specific treatments and interventions may vary.

Rosacea and Leaky Gut

Similar to other skin conditions, a leaky gut can affect rosacea by triggering systemic inflammation, immune dysregulation, and microbial imbalances. It is worthwhile to mention that chronic immune activation in rosacea occurs through the overactivation of T-cells, a type of white blood cell that we discussed in the *Psoriasis* section above. Overactive T-cells can attack skin cells, contributing to the inflammatory processes seen in rosacea.

Additionally, in rosacea, inflammation and immune responses can affect blood vessels, leading to visible blood vessels and flushing. This is part of the neurovascular response to immune stimuli.

Latest Research

Studies have shown that SIBO (Small Intestinal Bacterial Overgrowth) induced by a leaky gut could contribute to rosacea.

As noted earlier, SIBO is an overgrowth of bacteria in the small intestine, where relatively few bacteria are typically found. This overgrowth can disrupt normal digestion and nutrient absorption, leading to gastrointestinal symptoms like bloating, diarrhea, and abdominal pain. SIBO can contribute to rosacea through the mechanism described for other skin diseases: gut inflammation and immune response through inflammatory mediators. Additionally, bacteria involved in SIBO can release toxins that further exacerbate inflammation and contribute to skin conditions like rosacea.

Lastly, we will switch gears and look at how specific leaky gut-induced nutrient deficiencies affect our skin.

Nutrient Deficiencies in Leaky Gut and their Skin Manifestations

When your gut is leaky, it may not be able to fully absorb vitamins and minerals, leading to deficiencies that negatively impact your skin. Here's how specific deficiencies can affect you:

- ❖ *Dry, Flaky Skin*: Insufficient vitamin D and omega-3 fatty acids can result in dry, flaky, and itchy skin.
- ❖ *Slow Wound Healing*: A lack of vitamins D and E, as well as zinc, can slow the healing process for cuts, scrapes, and other skin wounds, increasing your risk of infections.
- ❖ *Skin Lesions and Irritation*: Zinc deficiency can lead to skin lesions, increased irritation, and a higher likelihood of developing inflammatory skin conditions.
- ❖ *Hair Loss*: Without enough zinc, you might experience hair loss, as zinc is essential for hair tissue growth and repair. It also helps maintain the integrity of oil glands around hair follicles, which is crucial for healthy hair.

❖ *Hyperpigmentation:* Insufficient vitamin B12 can lead to hyperpigmentation, causing dark patches on the skin.

Diagnosing Leaky Gut

Diagnosing leaky gut can be challenging, as its symptoms are often nonspecific and overlap with other conditions. However, several tests can help identify increased intestinal permeability:

Lactulose-Mannitol Test

This test measures the absorption of two sugar molecules, lactulose and mannitol, by measuring their urine levels after ingestion. Lactulose is larger and should not be easily absorbed, while mannitol is smaller and easily absorbed. Elevated levels of mannitol in the urine indicate good absorption and, by extension, a healthy intestinal lining. Low levels of lactulose indicate that the intestinal lining is intact and not overly permeable.

Elevated levels of lactulose in the urine can indicate increased intestinal permeability. A ratio of lactulose to mannitol in the urine is used to assess intestinal permeability. A higher ratio indicates increased intestinal permeability (leaky gut), while a normal or low ratio suggests normal intestinal function.

Zonulin

Zonulin is a protein that is viewed as a biomarker of gut permeability. It regulates tight junctions between intestinal cells, and elevated zonulin levels in the blood or stool indicate increased intestinal permeability.

Latest Research

Recent studies have hypothesized that zonulin may be a predictor of diabetes. Elevated zonulin levels are observed in type 1 and type 2 diabetes patients. They may be used to predict the onset and progression of diabetes and its related complications.

Comprehensive Stool Analysis

Multiple advanced stool tests are now available on the market. Most of them are easy to perform, as they are based on patients submitting stool specimens—this is done at home.

As mentioned earlier, our gut is home to trillions of microorganisms. A state-of-the-art technique called quantitative PCR is used to identify and measure them. This exact method identifies gut microorganisms by their genes. The quantity of microorganisms is essential. For example, a lower bacteria count is likely to make these bacteria a colonizer and thus not specifically harmful to the body. However, a high quantity of the same bacteria is likely to translate into an infection.

Microbiology components of a gut test:

- ❖ *Bacteria:* pathogenic, opportunistic, and beneficial bacteria are measured. Pathogenic bacteria indicate an infection if beyond a certain threshold in quantity. The presence of opportunistic bacteria may indicate a potential for infection or low-grade inflammation in some cases. Overgrowth of certain bacteria can point to functional disorders of the gut. An insufficient number of beneficial bacteria is concerning as well, as it may affect gut absorption and digestion of essential nutrients.

- *Parasites:* This section includes checking for worms and protozoa, one-cell organisms that may act as parasites. One of the biggest surprises for patients in the Western World is the presence of parasites in their stool in the absence of any recent or even remote exotic travel.

  Parasitic infections are unfortunately more common than one might expect, often linked to a leaky gut. Despite this, they are frequently overlooked by conventional medicine, especially when the symptoms presented are unrelated to gastrointestinal issues.

  A smoldering chronic parasitic infection can exacerbate your common skin issues, such as eczema and psoriasis, for example.

- *Viruses:* Cytomegalovirus and Epstein-Barr virus (EBV) are among the common viruses that are checked. You may have heard that EBV has been linked to chronic fatigue syndrome.

- *Fungi:* Candida species, as well as other fungi in stool, could significantly contribute to many medical conditions, including the skin, and be very hard to eradicate.

The other part of the comprehensive stool test is dedicated to measuring various gut health markers, such as the ones for digestion, inflammation, and immune response. These markers may show problems with pancreatic function or indicate the presence of inflammatory bowel disease, for example. They are extremely useful as starting points in the investigation of gut health. Some abnormal parameters may necessitate further workup, such as colonoscopy, for example.

Analysis of these markers, along with the microbiology results, helps establish a diagnosis of leaky gut and its degree. Most importantly, it helps create a treatment plan based on diet and supplemental support. A clear skin diet is first a gut-friendly diet.

CHAPTER 6

Hormones and Food Sensitivities

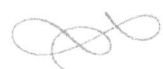

In this section, we will discuss how different hormones are affected by food sensitivities and how they impact our skin health. We will focus on insulin and insulin-like growth factor (IGF-1), hormones in dairy, stress hormones, sex hormones (testosterone, estrogen, progesterone), and thyroid hormones.

Insulin and Insulin-Like Growth Factor (IGF-1) and Skin Health

Insulin is vital for maintaining stable blood sugar levels. When insulin functions properly, it transports glucose into cells, providing them with the necessary energy. However, elevated insulin levels can increase sebum production, which in turn leads to clogged pores, aggravating acne.

Insulin-like Growth Factor (IGF-1) works alongside insulin to promote cell growth and regeneration. However, similar to insulin, elevated levels of IGF-1 cause overproduction of sebum and exacerbate acne.

Dairy and high-glycemic foods trigger both insulin and IGF-1.

Dairy contain IGF-1, which can further increase oil production and promote the development of acne. People with sensitivities to dairy products may experience worse skin conditions due to this hormonal disruption.

High-glycemic foods trigger insulin release and start the domino effect towards acne aggravation.

High stress can also increase insulin and IGF-1 production.

To keep insulin and IGF-1 levels balanced and maintain healthy skin, consider a low-glycemic diet and reduce dairy intake or switch to dairy alternatives.

Regular exercise helps regulate blood sugar levels and improve insulin sensitivity, positively impacting skin health.

Androgens: Testosterone and Dihydrotestosterone (DHT) and Skin Health

Androgens are male sex hormones that include testosterone and its potent derivative, dihydrotestosterone (DHT). While these hormones are produced in men and women, their levels and effects can differ significantly. In terms of the impact on the skin, androgens are essential in regulating sebum (oil) production, which is vital for maintaining healthy skin.

However, when androgen levels are too high, they can lead to excessive sebum production. This can clog pores and create an environment where acne-causing bacteria thrive, resulting in breakouts and oily skin.

Androgens also promote the growth and turnover of skin cells. While this is necessary for normal skin renewal and healing, an overabundance of skin cells combined with increased sebum production can clog pores. This clogging can lead to acne, as trapped oil and dead skin cells create an ideal breeding ground for bacteria.

How Food Sensitivities May Affect Androgen Levels

Food sensitivities can exacerbate the effects of androgens on the skin.

Let's explore two primary dietary culprits: dairy products and high-glycemic foods.

Dairy Products and High-Glycemic Diet

We have just discussed how dairy and high-glycemic foods increase insulin and insulin-like growth factor, IGF-1.

In women, insulin and IGF-1 increase the production of androgens, including testosterone, directly by stimulating the cells in the ovary to produce more androgens and indirectly through enzyme reactions involved in hormone production.

Yes, female ovaries do produce testosterone! Testosterone is important for sexual desire, bone health, and energy levels. So, in women, insulin and IGF-1 lead to an **increase** in testosterone production.

On the contrary, increased levels of insulin in men lead to insulin resistance, which in turn **decreases** the production of testosterone.

These hormonal imbalances have different manifestations in men and women.

Men may develop gynecomastia (breast tissue development), increased body fat, particularly in areas typical for female fat distribution (hips, thighs), reduced muscle mass, and decreased libido and sexual function.

Polycystic Ovary Syndrome (PCOS) in women is a mirror example of such imbalance, where insulin resistance results in increased testosterone production, contributing to symptoms like hirsutism (excessive hair growth), acne, and irregular menstrual cycles.

Estrogen and Skin Health

Estrogen is a female sex hormone mainly produced by the ovaries that helps regulate the menstrual cycle and is essential in the development of secondary female characteristics and in pregnancy.

Estrogens contribute to the following skin functions:

- ❖ *Collagen Production:* Estrogen boosts collagen production, which keeps your skin elastic and firm. More collagen means a fuller, more youthful look.

- *Hydration and Moisture:* Estrogen increases hyaluronic acid, which retains moisture in your skin. This helps keep your complexion smooth and hydrated.
- *Sebum Regulation:* Estrogen helps control the production of sebum. Balanced sebum levels prevent your skin from becoming too oily or too dry, reducing acne and other skin issues.
- *Skin Thickness:* Estrogen maintains your skin's thickness by encouraging cell growth and turnover, keeping your skin resilient and damage-resistant.
- *Anti-Inflammatory Properties:* Estrogen can reduce redness, swelling, and irritation, helping with conditions like rosacea and eczema.
- *Healing and Repair:* Higher estrogen levels speed up wound healing and repair of damaged skin tissue.
- *Pigmentation:* Estrogen affects melanocytes, the cells responsible for skin pigment, improving skin tone and reducing hyperpigmentation and age spots.

What Happens to Your Skin if There is Too Much Estrogen?

Like any imbalance, too much estrogen is not good for the skin and may cause the following skin issues:

- *Increased Skin Pigmentation:* Elevated estrogen levels can boost melanin production, leading to dark spots or melasma, often seen in pregnant women.
- *Increased Sebum Production:* High estrogen levels can cause your skin to become oilier, potentially leading to clogged pores and acne.

- **Vascular Changes:** High estrogen levels (relative to progesterone) can increase blood flow to your skin, causing a flushed appearance or more pronounced redness, which can worsen rosacea.
- **Altered Skin Healing:** Excess estrogen can disrupt your skin's normal healing processes, leading to irregular healing patterns or increased risk of certain skin conditions.

What Happens to Your Skin When There is Not Enough Estrogen?

When estrogen levels decline, especially during menopause, your skin can be affected in several ways:

- **Decreased Collagen:** Reduced collagen production makes your skin thinner and less elastic, causing more prominent fine lines and wrinkles.
- **Reduced Hydration:** Lower levels of hyaluronic acid result in drier skin, which can feel tight and flaky.
- **Increased Skin Sensitivity:** Your skin may become more prone to irritation and inflammation.
- **Sagging and Loss of Firmness:** Lower levels of elastin and collagen cause your skin to sag and lose its firmness.
- **Slower Healing:** Your skin's ability to heal and repair itself diminishes, making it more susceptible to damage.

To address these issues in post-menopausal women, estrogen replacement and topical estrogens are used.

How Food Sensitivities May Affect Your Estrogen Levels

As mentioned earlier, food sensitivities can trigger chronic inflammation and a leaky gut. Chronic inflammation and metabolic disruptions from food sensitivities can lead to weight gain and increased adipose (fat) tissue. Our fat tissue produces estrogen. Increased adiposity can result in higher estrogen levels, further contributing to hormonal imbalances. At the same time, chronic inflammation can affect estrogen metabolism in the liver, leading to a surplus of estrogen.

A leaky gut can impair the gut's ability to process and eliminate estrogens effectively, resulting in higher estrogen levels and hormonal imbalances. It also results in impaired nutrient absorption. Essential nutrients like B vitamins, magnesium, and zinc are critical for hormone synthesis and metabolism. Deficiencies in these nutrients can disrupt estrogen production and balance.

As noted earlier, certain food sensitivities, especially high-glycemic foods, can trigger insulin resistance. This can disrupt the balance of sex hormones, increasing androgen (testosterone) production, which can then be converted to estrogens in adipose tissue, elevating estrogen levels and causing hormonal imbalances.

How Estrogens in Food Affect Your Skin

Estrogens in Soy

Soy contains phytoestrogens, plant-derived compounds that can mimic estrogen in your body. For some, these can provide beneficial effects, especially for postmenopausal women. However, being sensitive to soy can lead to hormonal imbalances, affecting your skin by causing dryness, irritation, or worsening acne. See more about soy in *Chapter 8. Soy Sensitivity and Skin Conditions.*

Estrogens in Dairy

- ❖ *Natural Estrogens:* Milk contains natural animal estrogens like estrone (E1), estradiol (E2), and estriol (E3). These hormones are produced by the cows' ovaries, adrenal glands, and other tissues.
- ❖ *Synthetic Estrogens*: While not typically found in milk, synthetic hormones can sometimes be present due to hormone treatments in dairy cows. This can influence the hormone profile of the milk, although the direct impact on estrogen levels is debated.

   Milk is regulated to ensure safety and quality. The use of synthetic hormones like rBST is allowed in the U.S. but banned in the European Union, Canada, and other countries. Here are some definitions regarding the hormone levels in milk:

   Organic Milk: Produced without antibiotics, synthetic hormones, or pesticides.

   rBST-free Milk: Indicates that synthetic growth hormones were not used.

Synthetic estrogens in dairy can raise overall estrogen levels, potentially leading to hormonal imbalances and skin issues like increased oil production, clogged pores, and acne.

There is also increasing research regarding the effects of natural hormones in milk on puberty and cancer development. The data is inconclusive at this point.

Progesterone and Skin Health

Progesterone is a female sex hormone produced primarily by the ovaries. It plays a key role in regulating the menstrual cycle and maintaining pregnancy.

Progesterone also regulates sebum production. Fluctuations in progesterone can cause excessive or reduced sebum production, leading to acne or dryness.

Progesterone has anti-inflammatory properties that help soothe and calm your skin. It reduces redness, swelling, and irritation, promoting a clearer complexion.

During your menstrual cycle, progesterone levels fluctuate, peaking in the luteal phase (post-ovulation) and declining if pregnancy does not occur. These shifts can lead to premenstrual breakouts and changes in skin texture.

How Food Sensitivities May Affect Your Progesterone Levels

Food sensitivities can impact progesterone levels similarly to estrogen, stressing your adrenal glands and affecting their ability to produce adequate progesterone. Specific food sensitivities can impact progesterone levels by causing inflammation, hormonal imbalances, and gut health issues. Here are some common food sensitivities that can affect progesterone (you will see an overlap with estrogen.)

Gluten

Gluten sensitivity can cause inflammation and damage to the intestinal lining, leading to leaky gut syndrome. This increases systemic inflammation and disrupts hormonal balance, potentially reducing progesterone levels.

Dairy

Dairy sensitivity can increase inflammation and contribute to hormonal imbalances, particularly affecting the balance between estrogen and progesterone.

Soy

Soy contains phytoestrogens, which can mimic estrogen in the body. For individuals sensitive to soy, these compounds can disrupt the estrogen-progesterone balance, potentially leading to lower progesterone levels.

Sugar and High-Glycemic Foods

Sensitivity to high sugar intake can lead to insulin resistance and increased cortisol levels. This hormonal disruption can lower progesterone levels.

Alcohol

Alcohol sensitivity can affect liver function, which is crucial for hormone metabolism. Impaired liver function can disrupt the balance of estrogen and progesterone.

Processed Foods and Additives

Many processed foods contain additives, preservatives, and unhealthy fats that can trigger inflammation and disrupt gut health. This can affect the overall hormonal balance, including progesterone levels.

Thyroid Hormones and Skin Health

Thyroid hormones, primarily thyroxine (T4) and triiodothyronine (T3), are responsible for our energy levels, metabolic rate, and many other functions throughout the body.

When it comes to skin, thyroid hormones are responsible for various aspects of skin physiology:

- *Skin Cell Turnover and Repair*: Thyroid hormones stimulate the proliferation of keratinocytes, the primary cells in the epidermis, promoting healthy skin cell turnover and repair.
- *Wound Healing*: Adequate levels of thyroid hormones enhance the skin's ability to heal wounds by accelerating the repair processes.
- *Collagen Synthesis*: Thyroid hormones help regulate the production of collagen, a critical protein that provides structure and elasticity to the skin.
- *Skin Firmness*: Proper thyroid function maintains skin firmness and prevents sagging and wrinkles by supporting collagen integrity.
- *Sebum Production*: Thyroid hormones influence sebaceous gland activity. Balanced sebum production helps moisturize skin and prevents dryness or excessive oiliness.
- *Thermoregulation*: Thyroid hormones help maintain body temperature, which affects blood flow to the skin.

Proper circulation ensures adequate nutrient and oxygen supply to skin cells, promoting healthy skin.

- ❖ *Vasodilation:* These hormones can induce vasodilation, improving blood flow and nutrient delivery to the skin.
- ❖ *Hair Growth:* Thyroid hormones are crucial for the normal growth cycle of hair follicles. Imbalances can lead to hair thinning, loss, or changes in hair texture.
- ❖ *Pigmentation:* Thyroid hormones can affect melanocytes, the cells responsible for skin pigmentation. Abnormal thyroid levels can lead to changes in skin color, such as hyperpigmentation or paleness.

Thyroid Hormone Imbalance

- ❖ **Hypothyroidism**: This condition is characterized by low thyroid hormone levels and can lead to dry, rough, pale skin, hair thinning, and slower wound healing.
- ❖ **Hyperthyroidism**: High levels of thyroid hormones can result in warm, moist, and sometimes itchy skin, hair thinning, and increased sweating.

A few words about Iodine:

Iodine is essential for making thyroid hormones. Too little or too much Iodine can result in thyroid level imbalances.

- ❖ **Iodine deficiency leads to** hypothyroidism. If you are sensitive to iodine-rich foods like seafood, most dairy products, and iodized salt, then you may develop hypothyroidism.

❖ **Too much Iodine** can cause hyperthyroidism or thyroiditis, resulting in warm, moist skin, increased sweating, and itching.

How Food Sensitivities May Affect Thyroid Hormones

Food sensitivities can affect thyroid hormones through mechanisms involving inflammation, immune responses, and disruptions in gut health.

Food sensitivities can trigger autoimmune responses that target the thyroid gland, leading to conditions such as Hashimoto's thyroiditis (hypothyroidism) or Graves' disease (hyperthyroidism).

Inflammation and damage to the gut lining can impair the absorption of essential nutrients needed for thyroid function, such as iodine, selenium, zinc, and iron.

Food sensitivities can increase cortisol production due to chronic inflammation and stress on the body. Elevated cortisol levels can disrupt the balance of thyroid hormones by affecting the conversion of T4 to T3, the active form of thyroid hormone. So, stress definitely affects thyroid health!

Here are how specific foods can affect thyroid function:

Gluten

A very important cross-reactivity:

Certain foods that individuals may be sensitive to, like gluten, can cross-react with thyroid tissue, leading to an immune response against the thyroid.

Gluten sensitivity or celiac disease can lead to inflammation and autoimmune reactions that affect the thyroid gland. Studies show a higher prevalence of thyroid disorders among individuals with celiac disease. More about it in *Chapter 6. Gluten sensitivity and Skin Conditions*

Dairy

Sensitivity to dairy can cause inflammation and digestive issues that may interfere with nutrient absorption necessary for thyroid function.

Lactose intolerance can impair the absorption of thyroid medication, affecting the management of hypothyroidism.

Soy

Soy contains goitrogens, compounds that can interfere with thyroid hormone production. For individuals sensitive to soy, this interference can be more pronounced.

Studies indicate excessive soy consumption can affect thyroid function, particularly in individuals with existing thyroid conditions. More about it in *Chapter 8. Soy sensitivity and Skin Conditions.*

To optimize thyroid health, please eat nutrient-rich foods, including iodine (in moderation), selenium, zinc, and vitamins A and D.

Iodine sources are seafood, dairy products, and iodized salt.

Selenium sources are Brazil nuts, sunflower seeds, and fish.

Cortisol and Skin Health

Cortisol is often called the "stress hormone." It is released by the adrenal glands, which are situated above the kidneys. It helps the body respond to stress by raising blood sugar levels, enhancing glucose use in the brain, and increasing the availability of substances needed for tissue repair.

How Does Cortisol Work?

When you encounter a stressful situation, your body's fight-or-flight response is activated.

This response is regulated by the hypothalamic-pituitary-adrenal (HPA) axis, a complex system involving the hypothalamus (a part of your brain), the pituitary gland (also in your brain), and the adrenal glands. Here's a quick breakdown of how it works:

- ❖ The hypothalamus detects stress and releases corticotropin-releasing hormone (CRH).
- ❖ CRH signals the pituitary gland to release adrenocorticotropic hormone (ACTH).
- ❖ ACTH travels to the adrenal glands, prompting them to release cortisol into the bloodstream.
- ❖ Once released, cortisol helps prepare your body to handle the stressful situation by:
- Increasing blood sugar levels for quick energy.
- Enhancing brain function to improve focus and alertness.
- Suppressing non-essential functions, like digestion and reproduction, to prioritize dealing with the stressor.

Cortisol and Skin Health

When cortisol levels stay high for too long, they disrupt your skin's natural balance. Elevated cortisol can increase sebum (oil) production, leading to oily skin and acne. It can also weaken the skin's barrier, making it more susceptible to infections and irritants, worsening conditions like eczema and psoriasis.

How Food Sensitivities May Affect Cortisol Levels

Food sensitivities can increase cortisol production, further impacting skin health during acute and chronic stress situations.

Acute Stress

When your body sees certain foods as threats, it can trigger an immune response, increasing cortisol production to manage this perceived stress. This can lead to elevated cortisol levels even when there is no real danger.

High cortisol levels can stimulate the production of sebum. Excessive oil can clog pores, leading to breakouts and acne flare-ups.

Cortisol can trigger inflammatory responses affecting the whole body. In the skin, this inflammation may exacerbate conditions such as dermatitis, acne, and rosacea.

Chronic Stress

Food sensitivities can keep your body in a state of chronic stress, causing continuous cortisol production. This prolonged stress can exacerbate skin conditions like eczema and psoriasis and lead to additional issues such as fatigue and anxiety.

Cortisol-induced weakening of the immune system makes the skin more susceptible to infections and slows its healing process from injuries and inflammatory conditions.

Managing Stress and Cortisol for Better Skin Health

Here are common stress-reduction techniques:

Practicing yoga has been proven to reduce stress by promoting relaxation and mindfulness. Yoga postures, along with breathing exercises, can lower cortisol levels and enhance overall well-being.

Meditation soothes the mind and alleviates stress. It has been shown to lower cortisol levels and enhance emotional regulation.

Being physically active has been proven to reduce stress and lower cortisol levels. Walking, running, aerobics, pilates, and strength training can elevate mood and promote relaxation.

PART III

Common Food Sensitivities and Their Skin Effects

Now that you have learned what food sensitivities are and how they can affect the skin, let's look at specific foods and the diseases they may cause. Many concepts in this section should now be familiar, and some may be repetitious, as there is an overlap in both presentations and mechanisms of the effects of different food sensitivities on the skin.

CHAPTER 7

Gluten Sensitivity and Skin Conditions

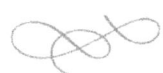

Gluten Sensitivity, Celiac Disease, Wheat Sensitivity, and Wheat Allergy: What's the Difference? Let's define gluten and its components.

Gliadin

Gliadin is a protein found in wheat and is one of the main components of gluten. In simple terms, gluten consists of two main proteins: gliadin and glutenin. Gliadin is responsible for many of the properties that make dough elastic and able to rise when baked.

Why is Gliadin Important?

For people with celiac disease, gliadin is particularly problematic. Here's why:

When someone with celiac disease eats foods containing gluten, their immune system mistakenly targets gliadin as a harmful substance. This sets off an immune response that damages the lining of the small intestine.

This immune response leads to inflammation and damage to the villi in the small intestine. Villi are small outpouchings in the intestinal lining that absorb nutrients from food. When they are damaged, nutrient absorption is impaired, leading to various symptoms and potential nutritional deficiencies.

Gliadin can be divided into several subtypes based on their amino acid sequences: alpha, beta, gamma, and omega-gliadin. Each subtype can trigger the immune response in celiac disease, but alpha-gliadin is the most reactive one.

Celiac Disease

Celiac disease is a serious autoimmune disorder where consuming gluten triggers an immune response that directly attacks your small intestine. In fact, small intestine involvement is the most important diagnostic factor in this disease.

Celiac disease has a genetic basis. There are 2 genes that are responsible for it, HLA-DQ2 and HLA-DQ8. These are specific genetic markers found on chromosome 6. People with celiac disease almost always have one or both markers.

- ❖ *HLA-DQ2:* This is the most common genetic marker found in about 95% of people with celiac disease.
- ❖ *HLA-DQ8:* This marker is less common but still significant, found in the remaining 5% of celiac cases.

In very rare cases, it is possible to have celiac disease in the absence of these genes.

The Inheritance Pattern

Celiac disease doesn't follow a simple inheritance pattern like some other genetic conditions. It's not as straightforward as saying that if your parents have it, you will too. However, having a first-degree relative (like a parent or sibling) with celiac disease increases your risk to about 1 in 10. This is because these genetic markers can be passed down through families.

While genetics are crucial, they are not the whole story. Not everyone with the HLA-DQ2 or HLA-DQ8 markers will develop celiac disease. A pioneer in this field, Dr. Alessio Fasano, discovered that for celiac disease to manifest, three factors are needed:

- *Trigger, such as gluten*
- *Genetic predisposition, such as the presence of HLA-DQ2 and/or HLA-DQ8 genes*
- *The presence of leaky gut.*

That may explain the fact that the prevalence of celiac genes in the general population is 1:35, but only 1:105 will develop a celiac disease.

Symptoms of Celiac Disease

Symptoms can be wide-ranging and severe, including the symptoms of IBS: abdominal pain and bloating, diarrhea or constipation, fatigue, weight loss, skin rashes (such as dermatitis herpetiformis), and joint pain.

Dermatitis Herpetiformis

Dermatitis Herpetiformis (DH) is a classic cutaneous manifestation of celiac disease. It is a chronic skin condition that causes intensely itchy and blistering skin eruptions. Thankfully, it affects only 10% of people with celiac disease.

DH usually shows up as clusters of small, itchy blisters and bumps. The elbows, knees, buttocks, and scalp are common spots. The itching can be so intense that scratching leads to secondary infections and scarring.

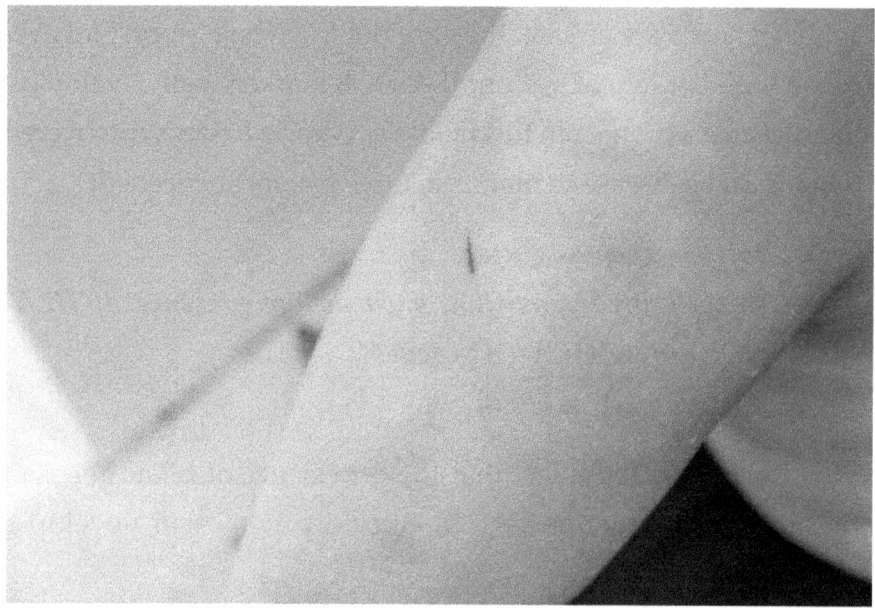

Figure 6.1 Dermatitis herpetiformis on the arm.

A clinical diagnosis of DH could be made, and a skin biopsy could confirm it by revealing deposits of immunoglobulin A (IgA) in the skin. Blood tests for celiac disease antibodies can also be helpful.

The main treatment for DH is a strict gluten-free diet. This reduces the antibodies that cause skin issues. Sometimes, medications like dapsone are prescribed to control itching and inflammation.

Diagnosis of Celiac Disease

The best way to diagnose celiac disease is through a blood test for IgA antibodies and a biopsy of the small intestine. Genetic testing can also help finalize the diagnosis.

Gluten Sensitivity

Gluten sensitivity, also known as non-celiac gluten sensitivity (NCGS), occurs when your body reacts to the gliadin component of gluten.

Interestingly, you don't have to have celiac genes to develop non-celiac sensitivity. Many researchers now consider NCGS a completely separate entity from celiac disease due to the lack of a common genetic and immune mechanism. Only 56% of people with NCGS have DQ2 or DQ8 genes.

Symptoms can include the same ones as in celiac disease but without a direct autoimmune assault on the small intestine. Also, dermatitis herpetiformis is almost never seen in NCGS.

Diagnosis is made through an elimination diet and clinical assessment. Regarding lab work, when suspecting NCGS, it is important to rule out celiac disease and wheat allergy or sensitivity.

Interesting Research

In a study by Dr. De Giorgio's group, many people with NCGS were found to have high levels of IgG antibodies against gliadin.

The study included 44 people with NCGS and 40 with celiac disease. Both groups followed a gluten-free diet for six months. The results showed that 93.2% of people with NCGS no longer had IgG antibodies after six months, indicating an excellent response to the diet. In contrast, only 40% of those with celiac disease saw a decrease in these antibodies.

The findings suggest that for people with NCGS, a strict gluten-free diet can lead to the disappearance of IgG antibodies and an improvement in symptoms.

Wheat Sensitivity

Non-celiac wheat sensitivity, or wheat intolerance, is when your body reacts to wheat but not necessarily to gluten. It is a broader sensitivity, as it entails sensitivities to other components of wheat with or without sensitivity to gluten.

Symptoms of wheat sensitivity often overlap with non-celiac gluten sensitivity and can include both intestinal and extraintestinal symptoms, including skin reactions.

Similarly to NCGS, wheat sensitivity may be diagnosed clinically and through an elimination diet. Also, IgG antibodies to wheat play a role in diagnosis.

Although this book is focused on food sensitivities and not on allergies, periodically, we will be discussing some allergies that are closely associated with the foods that are being featured. Here is a little about wheat allergy:

Wheat allergy is a very serious condition that happens with eating wheat products, or even accidentally inhaling wheat. Just like all allergies, the onset is quick, and reactions may vary from mild to severe, including anaphylaxis. The immune base of this allergy is production of IgE antibodies. The symptoms may include gastrointestinal, respiratory, and skin reactions.

How Gluten May Affect Your Skin

All three conditions: Celiac disease, non-celiac gluten sensitivity, and non-celiac wheat sensitivity can affect your skin, but the mechanisms and severity vary:

- ❖ Gluten triggers inflammation throughout your body.
- ❖ If you have eczema, gluten might cause more frequent and severe flare-ups characterized by red, inflamed, and itchy patches.
- ❖ Gluten can cause more redness, scaling, and itching in psoriasis.
- ❖ Additionally, chronic inflammation disrupts hormones like cortisol, androgens, and estrogens. As noted earlier, these hormones affect sebum production by stimulating acne, breaking down collagen (cortisol), and accelerating the onset of wrinkles and fine lines.
- ❖ Gluten sensitivity can impact your thyroid by molecular mimicry, leading to an autoimmune condition, such as

Hashimoto's thyroiditis. This can cause dry, rough skin, hair loss, and slow wound healing.

❖ Gluten is also known to cause leaky gut and gut microbiome dysbalance in affected individuals, resulting in skin issues associated with leaky gut.

❖ Here is a summary of the mechanism of gluten's impact on our skin.

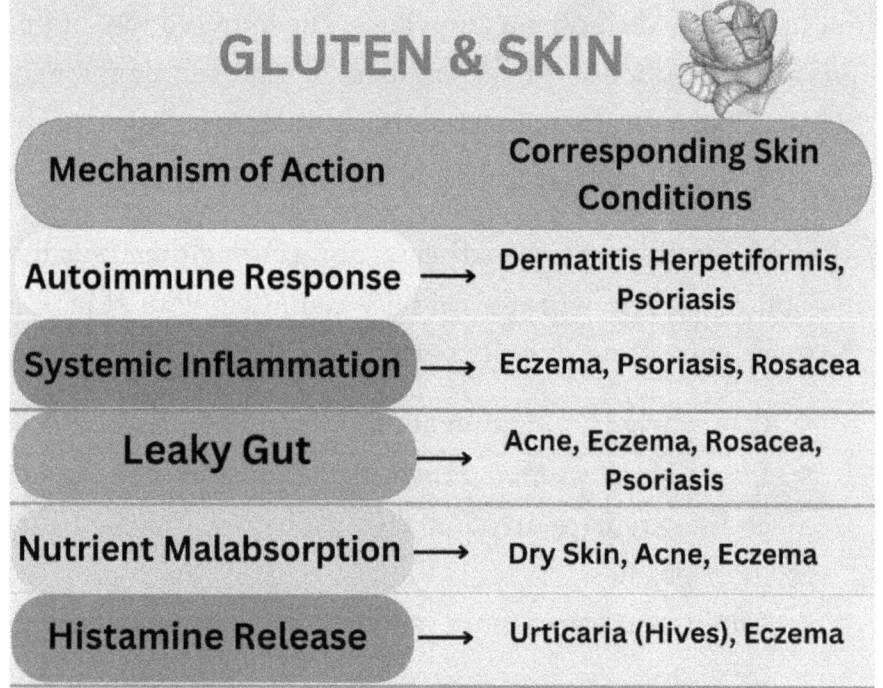

Figure 6.2 Mechanisms through which gluten may affect the skin.

Managing Gluten Sensitivity

The main treatment for gluten-related conditions is a strict gluten-free diet. Be sure to check food labels carefully and avoid cross-contamination.

Obvious Gluten-Rich Foods:

- ❖ Bread, pasta, cereals, and baked goods made from wheat, barley, and rye.

Hidden Sources of Gluten:

- ❖ *Soy Sauce:* Often contains wheat.
- ❖ *Gravies and Sauces:* Flour is frequently used as a thickener.
- ❖ *Processed Meats:* Some sausages, hot dogs, and deli meats can have gluten fillers.
- ❖ *Soups and Broths:* Gluten can lurk as a thickening agent or flavor enhancer.
- ❖ *Salad Dressings:* Some contain gluten for texture and flavor.
- ❖ *Beer and Malt Beverages:* Barley strikes again!

Gluten-Free Alternatives:

- ❖ *Bread and Pasta:* Choose gluten-free versions made from rice, corn, quinoa, or chickpeas.
- ❖ *Flours:* Try almond flour, coconut flour, or gluten-free all-purpose flour blends.
- ❖ *Soy Sauce Substitute:* Use tamari or coconut aminos.
- ❖ *Snacks:* Go for gluten-free crackers, pretzels, and chips.
- ❖ *Beer Alternatives:* Look for gluten-free beers or enjoy cider and wine.

- ❖ *Thickeners:* Use cornstarch or arrowroot powder instead of wheat flour.

Adopting a gluten-free diet is essential for those with celiac disease, non-celiac gluten sensitivity, or non-celiac wheat sensitivity. However, eliminating gluten-containing foods can sometimes result in nutrient deficiencies.

Here's a closer look at the potential deficiencies:

Common Nutrient Deficiencies When Going Gluten-Free

Fiber

- ❖ *Challenge:* Many gluten-containing grains, like wheat, barley, and rye, are high in fiber. A gluten-free diet can often lack sufficient fiber.
- ❖ *Solution:* Incorporate gluten-free whole grains such as quinoa, brown rice, millet, and gluten-free oats, as well as fruits, vegetables, legumes, nuts, and seeds.

Iron

- ❖ *Challenge:* Gluten-containing grains are often fortified with iron. Without these grains, there is a risk of iron deficiency, which can lead to anemia.
- ❖ *Solution:* Consume iron-rich foods like lean meats, poultry, fish, lentils, beans, spinach, and fortified gluten-free cereals. Pairing these with vitamin C-rich foods can enhance iron absorption.

Calcium and Vitamin D

- *Challenge*: Many gluten-free diets lack dairy products, which are primary sources of calcium and vitamin D.
- *Solution*: Include calcium-rich foods like leafy greens, almonds, fortified non-dairy milk, and yogurt. Ensure adequate vitamin D intake through fatty fish, fortified foods, and supplements if necessary.

B Vitamins

- *Challenge*: Gluten-containing foods, especially whole grains, are significant sources of B vitamins, including thiamin, riboflavin, niacin, and folate.
- *Solution*: Eat various gluten-free whole grains, nuts, seeds, meat, eggs, and leafy greens. Consider fortified gluten-free products and supplements if needed.

Working with a licensed nutritionist can create a meal plan tailored to your individual needs, preferences, and nutritional requirements, including recommending appropriate supplements.

Chapter 8
Dairy Sensitivity and Skin Conditions

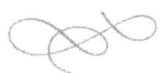

The main components of cow milk are casein and whey proteins. Casein protein makes up about 80% of the proteins in cow's milk and includes several subtypes.

Whey proteins have several subtypes, all of which can cause allergies and sensitivities. The most abundant one is beta-lactoglobulin. It is not found in human milk, which is why some individuals are more sensitive to cow's milk.

Let's discuss 3 conditions that are often used interchangeably despite having different immune mechanisms, different reactions and outcomes for our health. Those conditions are **dairy allergy, lactose intolerance and dairy sensitivity.**

Dairy Allergy

Dairy allergy is similar to other allergies in its fast onset and sometimes devastating symptoms. Dairy allergy works by the production of IgE antibodies. That means that drinking cow milk results in an almost immediate slew of symptoms, from hives to wheezing to anaphylaxis.

2.5% of children under 3 years of age are found to be allergic to milk, and they are usually diagnosed within the first year of life. Cow milk is the main culprit, but milk from other mammals, such as goats, sheep, etc., may also be implicated in this allergy.

Fortunately, most children outgrow this allergy, and it is very uncommon in adults.

The main management is avoiding dairy.

Lactose Intolerance

Lactose intolerance is a digestive disorder caused by the inability to digest lactose, the primary sugar in milk and dairy products. This condition occurs due to a deficiency in lactase, an enzyme produced in the small intestine that is necessary for breaking down lactose into glucose and galactose, which can be absorbed into the bloodstream.

When lactose is not properly digested, it passes into the colon, where it is fermented by bacteria. This fermentation process can cause a range of symptoms, including bloating, diarrhea, gas, abdominal pain, and nausea.

Symptoms typically occur within 30 minutes to 2 hours after consuming lactose-containing foods or beverages.

Lactose intolerance can be classified into several types based on its cause:

Primary Lactose Intolerance

The most common type is age-related lactose intolerance. It occurs due to a natural decline in the production of lactase, the enzyme responsible for breaking down lactose, as people age. This decline usually begins after childhood and continues into adulthood. In infants, high levels of lactase, an enzyme that helps digest lactose, are necessary to digest breast milk or formula. However, as children are weaned and their diets become more varied, the need for lactase decreases.

LCT is the key gene coding for lactase, an enzyme that helps digest lactose. It is identified during genetic testing.

Lactase persistence (ability to metabolize lactose into adulthood) is more common in populations with a long history of dairy farming and consumption, such as those of Northern European descent.

Lactase non-persistence (lactose intolerance) is more common in populations with less historical reliance on dairy, including many East Asian, African, and Middle Eastern groups.

> **Fun Fact:**
>
> Irish people are believed to have the best ability to metabolize lactose into adulthood, with only 5% of the Irish population being lactose intolerant.

Secondary Lactose Intolerance

This condition is caused by an illness, surgery, or injury affecting the small intestine, such as Crohn's disease, celiac disease, or gastroenteritis. Leaky gut and bacterial overgrowth have been implicated in this intolerance.

Congenital Lactase Deficiency

This rare inherited disorder occurs when babies are born with little or no lactase enzyme. This means they cannot tolerate breast milk and standard infant formulas, so they must be fed special lactose-free formulas.

How Lactose Intolerance is Diagnosed

Lactose intolerance can be diagnosed through several tests:

- ❖ *The Lactose Tolerance Test* measures serum glucose levels after ingesting a liquid containing high lactose levels. A smaller-than-expected rise in blood glucose levels after consuming lactose indicates that lactose is not being properly digested and absorbed, suggesting lactose intolerance.
- ❖ *Hydrogen Breath Test* measures the amount of hydrogen in the breath after consuming a lactose-rich beverage. If the body cannot properly digest lactose, the undigested lactose will be fermented by bacteria in the colon, producing hydrogen gas. Elevated levels of hydrogen in breath, measured at regular intervals after consuming the lactose solution, indicate lactose malabsorption and, therefore, lactose intolerance.

- ❖ *The Stool Acidity Test* is used primarily for infants and young children. It measures the amount of lactic acid in the stool. Normally, stool is not acidic, but the presence of lactic acid changes that. So, acidic stool (with a lower-than-normal pH) is abnormal and points towards an inability to metabolize lactose.

Managing Lactose Intolerance

- ❖ Reduce or eliminate lactose-containing foods depending on the severity of the lactose intolerance.
- ❖ Take over-the-counter lactase enzyme supplements to help digest lactose.
- ❖ Choose lactose-free dairy products that have the lactose removed or broken down.
- ❖ Ensure adequate calcium and vitamin D intake through lactose-free foods, supplements, or fortified products.

Dairy Sensitivity

Dairy sensitivity is a condition in which the immune system becomes sensitized to casein and whey milk proteins by producing antibodies and causing various delayed reactions.

Acne and Dairy Sensitivity

One of the most common skin issues linked to dairy sensitivity is acne. Dairy products can exacerbate acne through several mechanisms, depicted in this image.

// Dairy Sensitivity and Skin Conditions

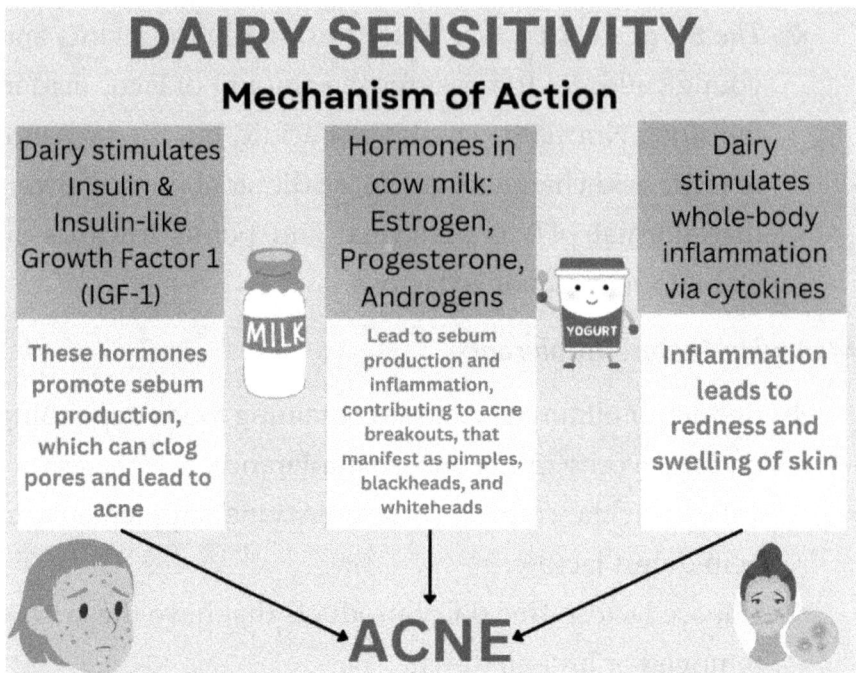

Figure 7.1 Mechanisms through which dairy may trigger and cause acne.

Interesting Fact:

Avoiding dairy products due to lactose intolerance may inadvertently lead to a lower frequency of acne in affected individuals.

Other Skin Conditions and Dairy Sensitivity

Dairy may cause or exacerbate many skin conditions through various mechanisms we studied earlier in this book. Here is a summary of the mechanism of dairy's impact on our skin.

THE CLEAR SKIN DIET

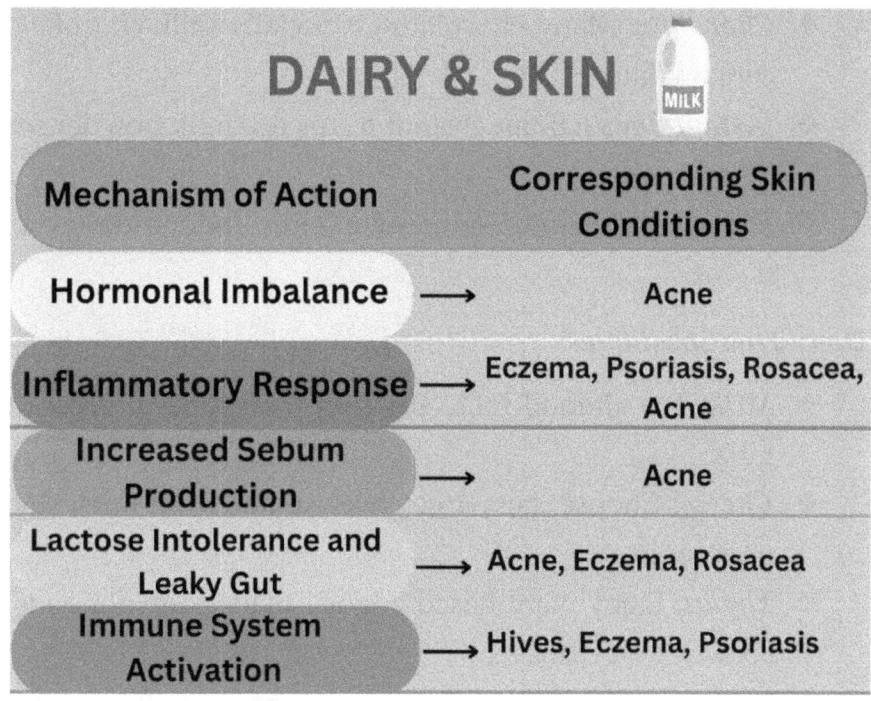

Figure 7.2 Mechanisms through which dairy may affect the skin.

Managing Dairy Sensitivity

Avoiding or decreasing dairy intake is the main strategy.

Obvious Dairy Food Sources:

❖ Milk, cheese, yogurt, butter, and cream.

Hidden Sources of Dairy:

❖ *Processed Foods:* Many packaged foods like chips, crackers, and cookies can contain dairy.

❖ *Salad Dressings:* Creamy dressings often have hidden dairy.

❖ *Baked Goods:* Cakes, pastries, and bread can contain butter or milk powder.

- ❖ **Chocolate:** Many chocolates, especially milk chocolate, contain dairy.
- ❖ **Instant Soups:** Some instant soups use milk powder for creaminess.
- ❖ **Breakfast Cereals:** Some cereals have added dairy for flavor.

Dairy-Free Substitutes:

- ❖ **Milk:** Try almond milk, soy milk, oat milk, or coconut milk.
- ❖ **Cheese:** Choose dairy-free cheese made from nuts, soy, or coconut.
- ❖ **Yogurt:** Enjoy plant-based yogurts made from almonds, coconuts, or cashews.
- ❖ **Butter:** Use coconut oil, olive oil, or dairy-free butter spreads.
- ❖ **Cream:** Substitute with coconut cream or cashew cream.
- ❖ **Ice Cream:** Indulge in dairy-free ice creams made from almond, coconut, or soy milk.

One of the challenges of going dairy-free is missing out on nutrients such as calcium, vitamin D, and B vitamins. Supplementation is often required.

CHAPTER 9

Soy Sensitivity and Skin Conditions

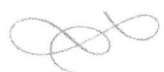

Soy is a dietary staple for many, particularly those following vegetarian or vegan lifestyles. It is obtained from the soybean plant, which is a type of legume. Soybeans are harvested from the plant pods and can be processed in various ways to produce a wide range of soy-based products, including soy milk, tofu, soy sauce, and soybean oil. The beans can also be fermented to create products like tempeh and miso. Rich in protein and essential nutrients, soy is beneficial for heart health and provides a plant-based protein source.

However, soy sensitivity can disrupt hormonal balance in the body, leading to various skin issues.

Phytoestrogens in Soy and Hormonal Disruption

As mentioned earlier, soy contains phytoestrogens, plant compounds that mimic estrogen in the body. For those with soy sensitivity, these phytoestrogens can disrupt the hormonal balance, particularly estrogen and progesterone levels, leading to increased oiliness, clogged pores, and acne breakouts. They can also exacerbate conditions like eczema by triggering inflammation and immune responses.

Yet, at the same time, phytoestrogens are beneficial for postmenopausal women in terms of decreasing osteoporosis and perimenopausal symptoms.

Soy and Thyroid Function

Soy can affect thyroid function in several ways, although its impact can vary based on individual health conditions and dietary habits.

Soy contains goitrogens, which are compounds that can interfere with the production of thyroid hormones. They do this by inhibiting the uptake of iodine, which is necessary for thyroid hormone production. This can potentially lead to goiter (an enlarged thyroid).

Soy is rich in isoflavones, a type of phytoestrogen. Some studies suggest that isoflavones may inhibit thyroid peroxidase (TPO), an enzyme involved in thyroid hormone synthesis. This inhibition can potentially reduce thyroid hormone levels.

Interestingly, adequate iodine intake can mitigate the thyroid-inhibiting effects of soy. In areas with sufficient iodine in the diet, the impact of soy on thyroid function is generally less significant. However, consuming large amounts of soy may pose a risk to thyroid health in individuals with low iodine intake.

Soy can also interfere with the absorption of synthetic thyroid hormones (like levothyroxine) used to treat hypothyroidism. People taking these medications are often advised to avoid consuming soy products close to the time they take their medication.

Overall, while moderate soy consumption is unlikely to significantly impact thyroid function in healthy individuals with adequate iodine intake, those with thyroid issues or on thyroid medication should consult with a healthcare provider to manage soy intake appropriately.

In the context of soy's impact on thyroid function, hypothyroidism triggered by soy may lead to dry skin and hair loss.

How Soy May Affect Your Skin

One of the most common skin issues directly linked to soy sensitivity is eczema. However, indirectly, through soy-induced thyroid and estrogen imbalance, other skin diseases, such as acne, rosacea, and psoriasis, could be impacted by soy.

Here is a summary of the mechanism of soy's impact on our skin.

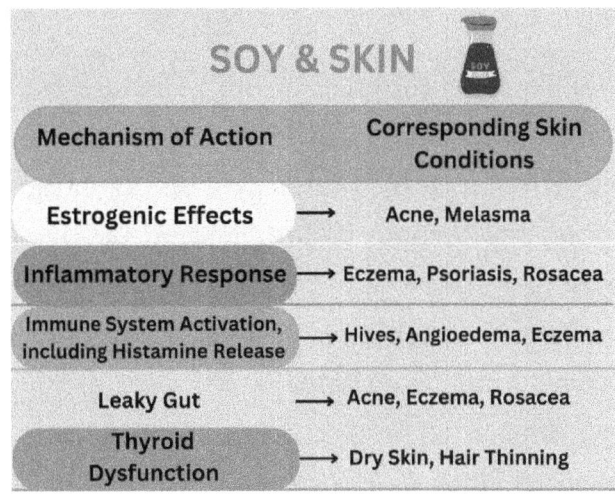

Figure 8.1 Mechanisms through which soy may affect the skin.

Managing Soy Sensitivity

The main treatment for soy sensitivity is adopting a soy-free diet.

Obvious Soy-Containing Foods:

- ❖ Soy sauce, tofu, tempeh, soy milk, edamame, and miso

Hidden Sources of Soy:

- ❖ *Processed Foods:* Many packaged foods like snacks, frozen meals, and meat substitutes contain soy.
- ❖ *Sauces and Dressings:* Teriyaki sauce and some salad dressings are soy based.
- ❖ *Baked Goods:* Some breads, pastries, and baked snacks use soy flour or soy lecithin.
- ❖ *Canned Soups:* May contain soy in broth and soup bases.
- ❖ *Protein Bars and Shakes:* Many use soy proteins as a key ingredient.
- ❖ *Vegetable Broth:* Sometimes contains soy, so always check the label.

Soy-Free Alternative:

- ❖ *Milk:* To substitute for soy milk, choose almond milk, coconut milk, oat milk, or rice milk.
- ❖ *Tofu Alternatives:* Use chickpea tofu or hemp tofu.
- ❖ *Sauces:* Try coconut aminos instead of soy sauce for a similar taste without the soy.
- ❖ *Snacks:* Choose soy-free snacks like veggie chips, fruit snacks, or nut-based bars.
- ❖ *Soy Proteins:* Go for pea protein, hemp protein, or brown rice protein instead of soy protein.

CHAPTER 10

Sugar Sensitivity and Skin Conditions

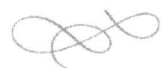

Of all the food sensitivities described in this book, this is probably the most dangerous for our general health. Although in this book we are focusing on skin manifestations of food sensitivities, it appears that the damage from sugar doesn't spare any organ system.

The situation is complicated by how ubiquitous sugar is in our daily diet, from healthy fruits to baked goods to processed meals.

We will examine how sugar affects the following conditions: acne, rosacea, seborrheic dermatitis, eczema, psoriasis, aging, skin infections, and hyperpigmentation.

Skin Diseases and Sugar

Acne and Sugar

Here is the mechanism through which sugar exacerbates acne:

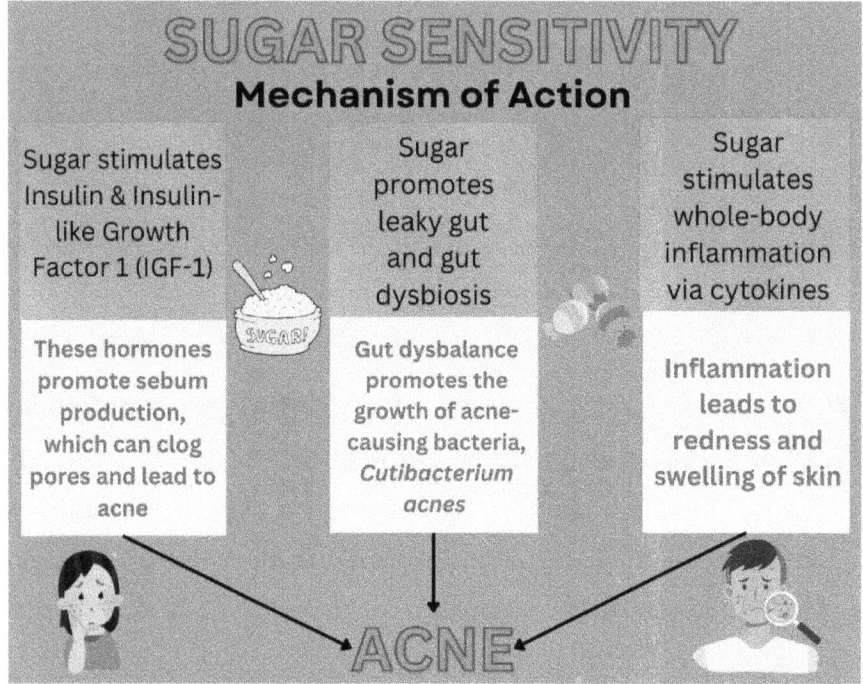

Figure 9.1 Mechanisms through which sugar may trigger and cause acne.

Interesting Research

Researchers have studied the Kitavan islanders of Papua New Guinea, who are known for having no acne. This phenomenon has been attributed to their traditional diet and lifestyle, which are vastly different from those in Western societies. The Kitavan diet is rich in tubers, fruits, fish, and coconut and lacks dairy, refined sugar, and processed foods. These dietary habits result in low glycemic index foods, which do not cause the insulin spikes associated with acne development in Western diets.

Additionally, the Kitavans have minimal exposure to Western influences and maintain a physically active lifestyle, which further supports their skin health. The absence of high-glycemic foods in their diet helps prevent hormonal fluctuations that can lead to excess oil production and clogged pores, thereby reducing the likelihood of acne.

This research highlights the potential impact of diet on skin health and suggests that adopting a diet low in high-glycemic foods and processed products may help manage or prevent acne.

Rosacea and Sugar

Sugar can exacerbate rosacea through several mechanisms involving inflammation, insulin spikes, and gut health. These mechanisms are similar to those that trigger acne.

Additionally, there are the following sugar-induced mechanisms:

- ❖ *Vasodilation:* High sugar-induced insulin spikes can lead to increased blood flow to the skin, worsening the flushing and redness.
- ❖ *Increased Sensitivity to Triggers:* Rosacea sufferers often have various triggers that can cause flare-ups, such as heat, stress, and certain foods. High sugar intake can make the skin more sensitive to these triggers. For example, sugar can amplify the body's response to heat

by increasing blood flow to the skin, leading to more severe flushing.
- ❖ **Yeast Infection:** High sugar consumption can negatively impact gut health by promoting the growth of harmful bacteria and yeast, such as Candida and Malassezia.

Sugar and Yeast Infection

A high-sugar diet can contribute to an overgrowth of yeast on the skin, particularly *Malassezia*. *Malassezia* is a naturally occurring yeast that thrives in oily areas of the skin. Still, when there is an excess of sugar in the body, it can promote the growth and activity of this yeast. Sugar can serve as a nutrient source for yeast, fueling its proliferation.

Impact on Seborrheic Dermatitis

Malassezia yeast, when present at high levels, plays a significant role in the development of seborrheic dermatitis. The breakdown of sebum into fatty acids by this yeast can irritate the skin, leading to the characteristic inflammation, redness, and flaky skin. A diet high in sugar can exacerbate this condition by encouraging yeast overgrowth, thereby triggering more severe symptoms of seborrheic dermatitis.

Rosacea and Yeast Interaction

While rosacea is primarily driven by factors such as vascular instability and immune system dysregulation, yeast overgrowth—possibly exacerbated by a high-sugar diet—can contribute to flare-ups, especially in individuals who have both rosacea and seborrheic dermatitis. The increased presence of

Malassezia can worsen the inflammation and redness seen in rosacea, leading to more persistent or severe symptoms.

Antifungal topical treatments are used to treat Malassezia species.

Eczema and Psoriasis and Sugar

Both eczema and psoriasis can be aggravated by inflammation triggered by sugar through the secretion of inflammatory cytokines. When sugar is consumed in excess, it can lead to spikes in blood glucose levels, which in turn can activate inflammatory pathways within the body.

In eczema, this heightened inflammatory state can increase itching, redness, and skin barrier dysfunction, while in psoriasis, it can lead to the rapid proliferation of skin cells, worsening the formation of thick, scaly plaques. By fueling these inflammatory processes, high sugar intake can make managing these chronic skin conditions more challenging.

Aging and Sugar (Glycation)

Let's talk about how sugar can age your skin through a process called glycation. Glycation happens when sugar molecules (like glucose and fructose) bind to proteins or fats in your body. This results in the formation of harmful molecules called advanced glycation end products (AGEs). As you get older, AGEs build up in tissues, especially where long-lived proteins like collagen and elastin are present.

AGEs' Impact on Your Skin

- Collagen is a protein in connective tissues, including skin, bones, tendons, ligaments, and cartilage, which keeps your skin firm and strong. AGEs make collagen fibers stiff and brittle, reducing your skin's ability to bounce back and leading to sagging and wrinkles.
- Elastin is another key protein in connective tissues that allows them to stretch and recoil, providing elasticity and resilience to structures such as skin, blood vessels, and lungs. Elastin allows your skin to stretch and recoil. When damaged by AGEs, elastin loses its flexibility, causing fine lines and deeper wrinkles. The stiffening of collagen and elastin fibers means your skin can't maintain its shape and firmness, making it more prone to wrinkles and sagging.
- AGEs activate receptors called RAGE on cells, triggering inflammation. This chronic low-level inflammation speeds up aging and further damages your skin.
- AGEs damage fibroblasts, the cells that produce collagen and elastin. This slows down your skin's ability to repair itself, making it more vulnerable to aging and damage.
- AGEs generate free radicals, leading to oxidative stress. This damages skin cells, proteins, and lipids, worsening skin aging.
- AGEs can dehydrate the skin, leading to dryness and a lackluster appearance.

Telomere Length and Sugar

Telomeres are protective caps at the ends of chromosomes that shorten with age. Research suggests that high sugar intake can accelerate the shortening of telomeres, contributing to aging and age-related diseases.

More specifically, high sugar intake leads to oxidative stress and inflammation, which accelerate the shortening of telomeres. As telomeres shorten, cells lose their ability to divide and function properly, leading to cellular aging and declining skin health.

Accelerated aging due to shortened telomeres can manifest as wrinkles, loss of skin elasticity, and a dull complexion.

Skin Infections and Sugar

Chronically elevated glucose predisposes us to infections, weakening our body's ability to protect us from bacteria, viruses, and fungi. This is why the rate and severity of infections in people with diabetes are higher.

Imagine walking on the beach barefoot, enjoying the scenery, and then stepping on a small piece of glass. If you are healthy, you may get away with a painful scrape and soon forget about it. If you have diabetes or even prediabetes, this tiny cut is more likely to get infected, with infection propagating higher on your foot and even resulting in a foot amputation. It sounds dramatic, but it is not an uncommon scenario at the Diabetes Clinic.

Hyperpigmentation and Sugar

Insulin resistance and high insulin levels, often a result of high sugar consumption, can lead to hyperpigmentation conditions like acanthosis nigricans (dark, velvety patches of skin), melasma, and post-inflammatory hyperpigmentation.

High-sugar diets can indirectly increase melanin production through hormonal and inflammatory pathways. Melanin is a natural pigment produced by cells called melanocytes in the skin, hair, and eyes, responsible for giving them their color. It also provides protection against the sun's ultraviolet (UV) radiation by absorbing and dissipating harmful rays. The overproduction of melanin leads to darker patches on the skin, particularly in areas prone to friction or sun exposure.

Let's look at these hyperpigmentation disorders:

Acanthosis Nigricans

Acanthosis nigricans is marked by dark, velvety patches of skin, typically in body folds and creases. It is often associated with insulin resistance and high insulin levels, and that is why it is more common in people with diabetes.

Melasma

Melasma is characterized by brown or gray-brown patches on the skin, often due to hormonal changes and sun exposure. It is most prominent on the face but occasionally can be seen on the neck, arms, and, less commonly, on the trunk. The most affected areas on the face are the sides of the cheeks / in front of the ears and an area above the lip, which may give the appearance of a mustache. High sugar intake can influence hormonal balance by exacerbating melasma.

Post-Inflammatory Hyperpigmentation (PIH)

As mentioned earlier, high sugar intake stimulates melanocytes to produce melanin. Due to the whole-body inflammation caused by high glucose, a minor skin injury or skin-picking habit in acne sufferers may lead to darker, scarred patches that are very hard to eradicate. This condition is manifested as dark and more pronounced scars.

Here is a summary of the mechanism of sugar's impact on our skin.

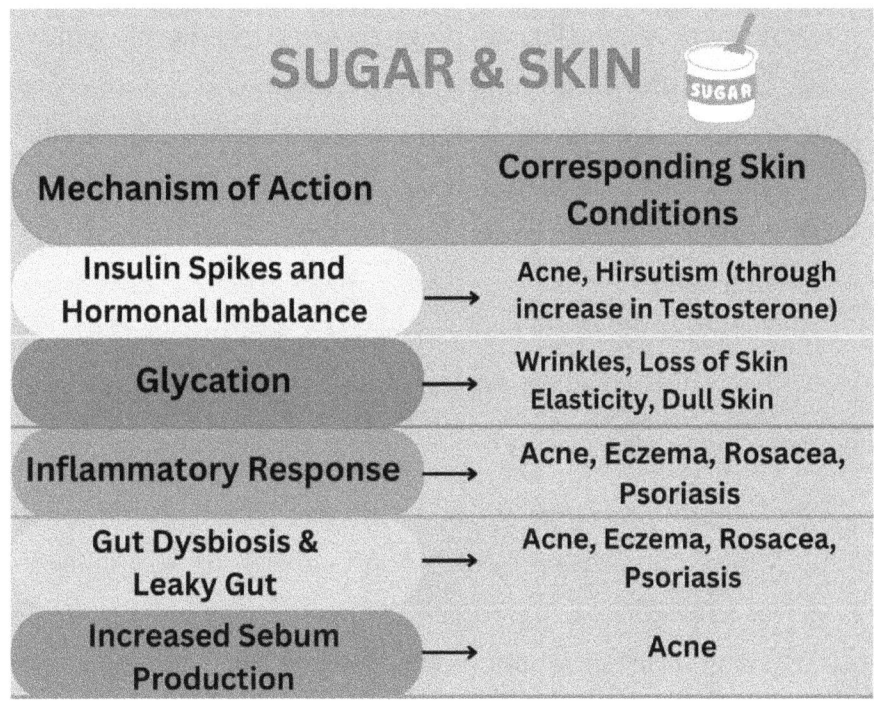

Figure 9.2 Mechanisms through which sugar may affect the skin.

Managing Sugar Sensitivity

It may not be completely realistic for some to eradicate all sugar from their daily diets, but decreasing the overall amount of sugar will benefit us on every level.

Obvious High-Sugar Foods:

- Candy, cakes, cookies, soda, and ice cream

Hidden Sources of Sugar:

- *Condiments:* Ketchup, barbecue sauce, and salad dressings
- *Bread and Baked Goods:* Even savory items like bread and rolls can have hidden sugar.
- *Yogurt:* Many flavored yogurts are packed with sugar.
- *Cereal and Granola:* Breakfast cereals and granola often contain significant amounts of sugar and, in reality, should be considered desserts.
- *Sauces and Marinades:* Pasta sauces, stir-fry sauces, and marinades.
- *Processed Foods:* Many packaged and processed foods have hidden sugar for flavor and preservation.

Healthy Sugar Alternatives:

- *Natural Sweeteners:* Use stevia or monk fruit in moderation, as these sweeteners don't spike your insulin levels as sugar does.
- *Fresh Fruits:* Satisfy your sweet tooth with naturally sweet fruits like berries, apples, and oranges.
- *Spices and Extracts:* Add flavor with cinnamon, vanilla extract, or almond extract instead of sugar.

- ❖ *Healthy Snacks:* Choose nuts, seeds, and unsweetened yogurt for a nutritious snack.
- ❖ *Beverages:* Choose water, herbal teas, or sparkling water with a splash of lemon or lime instead of sugary drinks.

Beware of Sugar Substitutes

While sugar substitutes might seem like a good idea, many can harm your health. Artificial sweeteners like aspartame, saccharin, erythritol and sucralose can cause digestive issues, disrupt gut bacteria, and even increase cravings for sweet foods. More data is coming out pointing towards the potential carcinogenic effects of artificial sweeteners.

Here is the summary of recent (2023) recommendation from the World Health Organization:

The World Health Organization (WHO) advises against using non-sugar sweeteners (NSS) for weight control or reducing noncommunicable disease risks, as they offer no long-term benefits and may increase risks of type 2 diabetes, cardiovascular diseases, and mortality. WHO recommends reducing dietary sweetness, including both free sugars and NSS, and consuming natural sugars from foods like fruit. This guideline applies to everyone except those with diabetes and includes all synthetic and naturally occurring NSS in foods and beverages. It excludes personal care products with NSS and low-calorie sugars. This recommendation is part of WHO's efforts to promote healthy diets and reduce disease risks worldwide.

Let's look at the popular artificial sweeteners:

Aspartame (Equal, NutraSweet)

Aspartame is 200 times sweeter than sugar.

The World Health Organization classified aspartame as a "possible carcinogen." High consumption of aspartame results in a 15% higher risk of developing cancers such as breast, endometrial, colon, stomach, and prostate cancers. However, this association does not confirm that aspartame directly causes cancer, as other factors might contribute to the increased risk.

Additionally, the long-term effects of aspartame consumption have been linked to obesity, diabetes, early menstruation, mood disorders, mental stress, and depression.

Saccharin (Sweet'N Low)

Saccharin is an artificial sweetener 200-700 times sweeter than sugar. It has been associated with several potential health risks, such as bladder cancer in rats, liver and kidney damage at high doses, and saccharin sensitivity and allergy reactions.

Erythritol (Swerve)

Erythritol is a sugar alcohol that is less sweet than sugar. In addition to its impact on gastrointestinal health, erythritol has been linked to heart attacks and strokes.

Sucralose (Splenda)

Sucralose is 600 times sweeter than sugar. Sucralose has been linked to leaky gut and DNA damage, predisposing habitual users to cancers.

CHAPTER 11

Egg Sensitivity and Skin Conditions

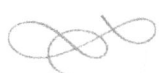

While some of the foods we have discussed so far, such as sugar, are questionable in their nutritional value, eggs, on the other hand, are filled with nutrients.

Facts About Eggs

- ❖ Eggs contain high-quality protein, vitamins (such as B12, D, A, and E), minerals (like selenium and phosphorus), and essential fatty acids.
- ❖ The color of an eggshell (white or brown) is determined by the breed of the hen. Nutritionally, there is no difference between white and brown eggs.
- ❖ Eggs have a relatively long shelf life when stored properly. Refrigerated eggs can last for about 3-5 weeks.
- ❖ Eggs contain cholesterol, primarily in the yolk. However, recent research suggests that eggs' dietary cholesterol minimally impacts most people's blood cholesterol levels.

- Organic eggs come from hens fed organic feed and not given antibiotics or hormones.
- Free-range eggs come from hens that have access to the outdoors. Both types are often considered more humane and environmentally friendly.
- A simple way to test egg freshness is to place it in a bowl of water. Fresh eggs will sink to the bottom and lie flat, while older eggs will stand upright or float due to the increased size of the air cell inside.
- Eggs hold cultural and symbolic significance in many traditions, such as Easter eggs in Christianity and eggs used in various fertility and creation myths worldwide.
- Many people think yolks are more allergenic than egg whites when it comes to egg allergies and sensitivities, but that is not true. Egg whites are more likely to cause a reaction.
- The proteins in egg whites, such as ovalbumin, ovomucoid, ovotransferrin, egg white lysozyme, and ovomucin, are more likely to trigger allergic reactions. Egg yolks also contain proteins, but they are generally less allergenic than those found in the whites.

Skin Diseases and Eggs

Here is a summary of the mechanism of eggs' impact on our skin.

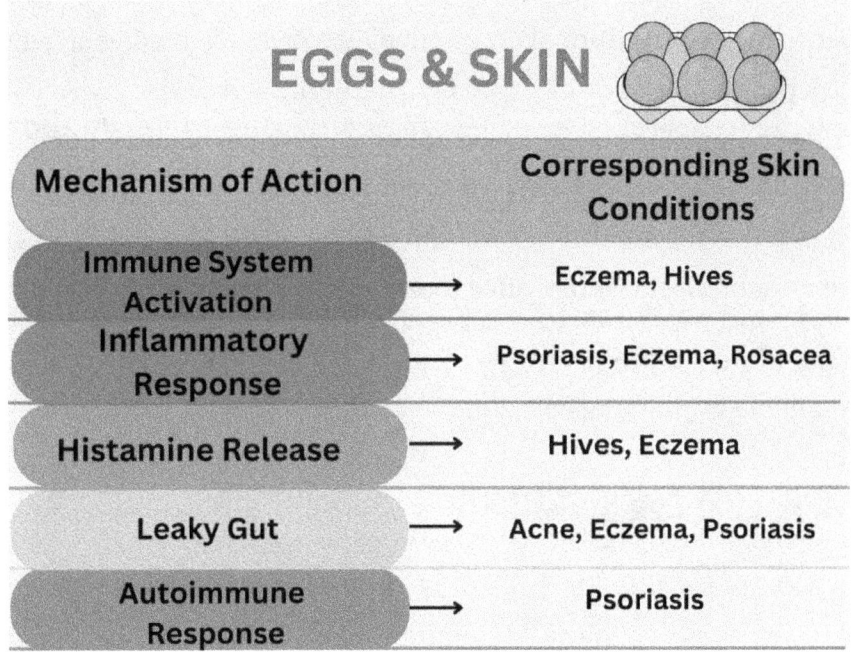

Figure 10.1 Mechanisms through which eggs may affect the skin.

Cross-Reactivity Between Egg Allergies and Flu Vaccines

Definition of Cross-Reactivity

Cross-reactivity happens when an individual's immune system reacts to proteins in one substance (e.g., a specific food or pollen) and mistakenly recognizes similar proteins in another substance as the same allergen, triggering an allergic reaction. It occurs due to the similarity in the protein structure of 2 different substances. The immune system produces IgE immunoglobulin to one substance, and due to similarity responds to the other similar substance, as well.

Cross-reactivity between egg and flu vaccines is important because most traditional flu vaccines are produced using an egg-based manufacturing process where the virus is grown in chicken eggs. This can introduce egg proteins, such as ovalbumin, into the vaccine. Unfortunately, that could be extremely dangerous for an individual with an egg allergy, as they can go into anaphylactic shock after receiving a flu vaccine.

Thankfully, there are now recombinant egg-free flu vaccines available on the market.

Managing Egg Sensitivity

If you are sensitive to eggs, it is important to find out whether you are sensitive to the egg white or yolk or both, as it will help you cut out only the component of the egg you are sensitive to. A food sensitivity test helps in distinguishing these two sensitivities (see *Chapter 20. Testing for Food Sensitivities*).

Obvious Egg-Containing Foods:

- ❖ Scrambled eggs, omelets, quiches, and baked goods

Hidden Sources of Eggs:

- ❖ *Processed Foods:* Many packaged foods like snacks and frozen meals
- ❖ *Sauces and Dressings:* Mayonnaise, hollandaise, and some salad dressings
- ❖ Bread and Baked Goods: Some bread and rolls

- Pasta: Fresh pasta
- Marshmallows and Meringues are made from egg whites.
- Battered and Breaded Foods: Coatings often use eggs as a binding agent.

Egg-Free Alternatives:

- *Baking Substitutes:* Use flaxseed meal or chia seeds mixed with water, applesauce, mashed bananas, or commercial egg replacers in your baking recipes.
- *Scramble Alternatives:* Try tofu scramble seasoned with turmeric and nutritional yeast for an egg-free breakfast.
- *Mayonnaise:* Choose egg-free mayo made from aquafaba or vegan options.
- *Egg-Free Pasta:* Look for pasta made without eggs, such as rice pasta or chickpea pasta.
- *Breading and Battering:* Use a mixture of flour and water or plant-based milk as a binder instead of eggs.

Are Commercial Egg Substitutes Safe?

Many commercial egg substitutes contain egg whites. The yolks are removed to decrease cholesterol and calories. Remember that it is the egg whites that are the most allergenic, so it is essential that you avoid these products if you have an allergy or sensitivity to egg whites.

CHAPTER 12

Nuts and Seeds Sensitivity and Skin Conditions

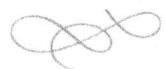

Facts About Nuts and Seeds

Just like eggs, nuts and seeds are highly nutritious and packed with healthy fats, proteins, vitamins, and minerals.

While an allergist may be well-informed about the difference between nut allergies and sensitivities, the public often uses them interchangeably despite the fact that they represent two different issues.

Since nut allergies are so common and comprise a high percentage of severe allergic reactions, including anaphylaxis, let's talk about them.

Peanuts are considered the most allergenic "nut." "However, peanuts are not real nuts, as they belong to the legume family. For reference, other members of the legume family are beans, lentils, peas, chickpeas, soybeans, and alfalfa.

Although there can be cross-reactivity between peanuts and other members of the legume family, it is relatively uncommon. The incidence of peanut allergies varies by region and population, but it has been increasing in many parts of the world.

Peanuts

- ❖ In the United States, peanut allergies affect approximately 2.5% of children. The prevalence has risen, with a significant increase observed over the past few decades.
- ❖ While peanut allergies are more common in children, they can persist into adulthood. About 1-2% of adults in the U.S. are estimated to have a peanut allergy.
- ❖ The prevalence of peanut allergies varies globally. In some Western countries, such as the United Kingdom, Australia, and Canada, the rates are similar to those in the U.S. However, the prevalence is generally lower in Asian countries, although it is increasing as Western dietary habits spread.
- ❖ Some studies suggest that peanut allergies are slightly more common in boys than in girls during childhood. However, this gender difference tends to equalize in adulthood.
- ❖ Risk factors for developing peanut allergies include a family history of allergies, having other allergies or atopic conditions (such as eczema or asthma), and possibly delayed introduction of peanuts into the diet.
- ❖ Recent research indicates that early introduction of peanuts into the diet of infants (around 4-6 months) who are at high risk for allergies (due to severe eczema or egg

allergy) can significantly reduce the risk of developing a peanut allergy. This has led to updated guidelines in several countries.

Tree Nuts

The next allergenic group after peanuts is tree nuts. The most common members of the tree nut family are almonds, walnuts, cashews, pecans, pistachios, hazelnuts, Brazil nuts, macadamia nuts, pine nuts and chestnuts.

Cross-Reactivity: Pollen-Food Syndrome or Oral Allergy Syndrome (OAS)

Oral allergy syndrome (OAS) symptoms typically occur in the mouth or throat after consuming certain foods like nuts, raw vegetables, or fruits, particularly in individuals who are allergic to specific pollens. These symptoms may include itching and tingling in the mouth, lips, throat, and sometimes ears immediately after eating the offending food. Mild swelling of the lips, tongue, and throat can also occur. Throat tightening, difficulty swallowing, and anaphylaxis are less common.

Here are examples of paired allergies in OAS involving peanuts and tree nuts:

- ❖ Birch pollen allergy can cause reactions to hazelnuts, walnuts, almonds, peanuts, apples, carrots, and celery.
- ❖ Grass Pollen can cause allergies to peanuts, peaches, celery, tomatoes, melons, and oranges.

- ❖ Mugwort pollen allergy can cross-react with sunflower seeds, peanuts, celery, carrots, and spices like coriander and parsley.
- ❖ Latex-Fruit Syndrome: Individuals allergic to latex may react to chestnuts, bananas, avocados, and kiwis because of similar proteins in latex and these foods.
- ❖ Tree Nut Cross-Reactivity: Allergic reactions to one type of tree nut (e.g., walnuts) can sometimes lead to reactions to other tree nuts (e.g., pecans) due to protein similarities.

Seeds

Seed allergies and sensitivities are less common than the ones to peanuts or tree nuts but are significant and can be severe.

The most common seed that people are allergic to is sesame. Other potentially allergenic seeds are sunflower, poppy, and mustard seeds.

The prevalence of sesame allergy, for instance, is estimated to be around 0.1-0.2% of the population in some countries.

Another example of cross-reactivity occurs when people with sesame seed allergies react to poppy seeds or sunflower seeds due to similar protein structures.

Symptoms of seed allergies can range from mild to severe. They may include hives, itching, swelling of the lips, face, or throat, abdominal pain, nausea, vomiting, diarrhea, and, in severe cases, anaphylaxis.

Skin Diseases and Nuts and Seeds

Here is the summary of the mechanism of nuts and seeds' impact on our skin.

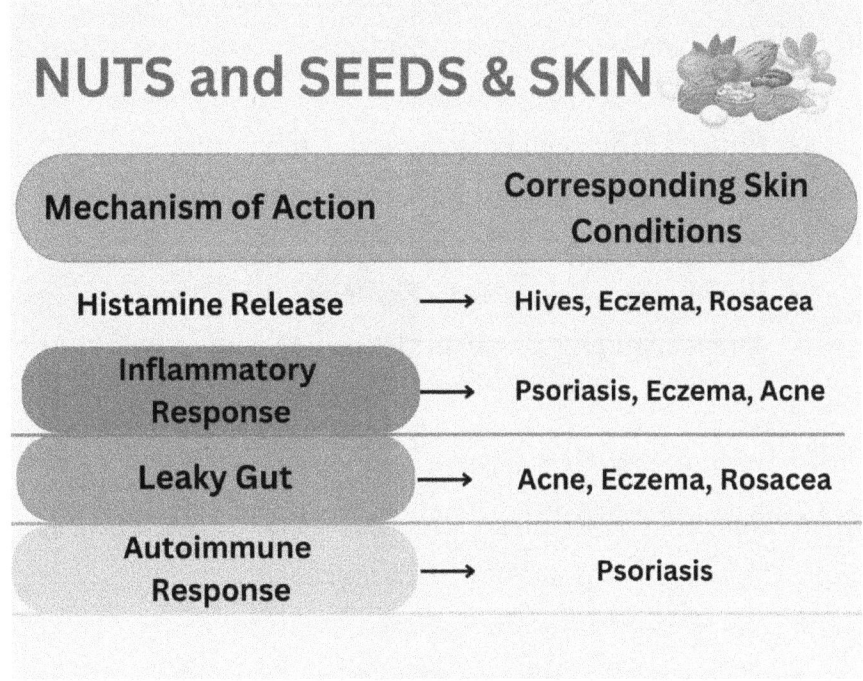

Figure 11.1 Mechanisms through which nuts and seeds may affect the skin.

Managing Nuts and Seeds Sensitivity

Avoidance of trigger nuts and seeds in the diet is the key.

Obvious Food Sources of Nuts and Seeds:

- ❖ Peanuts, and tree nuts: raw, roasted salted, unsalted, with honey, and other add-ons.
- ❖ Seed Butters

Hidden Sources of Nut and Seeds:

- ❖ *Processed Foods:* Many packaged snacks, granola bars, and protein bars
- ❖ *Baked Goods:* Muffins, breads, and pastries
- ❖ *Salad Dressings:* Some dressings and sauces use nuts or seeds for texture and flavor.
- ❖ *Pesto:* Traditional pesto contains pine nuts.
- ❖ *Cereals and Granolas:* Many breakfast cereals and granolas contain nuts or seeds.
- ❖ *Vegan and Vegetarian Products:* Nut-based cheeses, spreads, and meat substitutes can be loaded with nuts or seeds.

Nut-Free and Seed-Free Alternatives:

- ❖ *Baking Substitutes:* Use oat flour or coconut flour instead of almond flour in recipes.
- ❖ *Nut-Free Snacks*: Choose seedless dried fruits, popcorn, or vegetable chips.
- ❖ *Nut-Free Milks:* Choose rice milk, oat milk, or hemp milk instead of almond or cashew milk.

CHAPTER 13

Caffeine Sensitivity and Skin Conditions

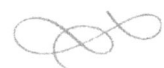

Many people think of reacting to caffeine in terms of feeling nervous, jittery, anxious, or developing a high heart rate and insomnia. These effects may be observed with a small to average amount of caffeine in sensitive people or too much caffeine in an average person.

However, in this book about food sensitivities and its effects on skin, we are discussing the effects of caffeine on your skin. These effects may or may not be accompanied by neurological symptoms.

You may be sensitive to caffeine without even knowing it. For example, you can develop a flare-up of eczema several hours after caffeine intake while not developing any jitters, elevated heart rate, and other neurological symptoms.

Mechanism of Caffeine Sensitivity

Let's start with definitions:

Caffeine is a natural stimulant found in the leaves, seeds, or fruits of more than 60 plants, including coffee beans, tea leaves, cacao pods, and kola nuts.

Caffeine works primarily by blocking the action of adenosine, a neurotransmitter that promotes sleep and relaxation. By inhibiting adenosine, caffeine increases the production of neurotransmitters like dopamine and norepinephrine, leading to increased energy and alertness. It can also boost metabolic rate and enhance physical performance by mobilizing fatty acids from the fat tissues and increasing adrenaline levels in the blood.

Genetics of Caffeine Sensitivity

Several genes influence how the body processes and responds to caffeine.

The main one is CYP1A2, an enzyme responsible for metabolizing caffeine in the liver.

Based on your genetic variant of CYP1A2, you could be a fast, slow, or average caffeine "metabolizer."

If you are a "fast metabolizer," you have an active version of this enzyme. It means that caffeine is broken down and cleared from your system faster than average, reducing the duration of its stimulating effects. You can drink several cups of coffee with minimal to no effects. You may also require more caffeine to achieve the desired stimulating effects.

If you are a "slow metabolizer," you have a more sluggish enzyme, leading to a slower caffeine metabolism. In "slow metabolizers," caffeine stays in the system longer, prolonging its effects and increasing the likelihood of side effects such as jitteriness, insomnia, and increased heart rate.

In general, slow metabolizers are more sensitive to caffeine's effects. They may experience stronger and longer-lasting stimulation and are at a higher risk of adverse effects even at lower doses of caffeine.

Typically, the half-life of caffeine (the time it takes for the body to eliminate half of the caffeine) for "fast metabolizers" ranges from 2.5 to 4.5 hours.

For "slow metabolizers," the half-life of caffeine can extend to 8 hours or more.

It has been shown that "slow metabolizers "who drank four or more cups of coffee per day have a significantly higher risk of nonfatal heart attack compared to non-coffee drinkers. Specifically, the risk was 64% higher for slow metabolizers.

In contrast, there is no increased risk of heart attack with higher coffee consumption in "fast metabolizers." In fact, moderate (1-3 cups) coffee consumption has been shown to be associated with a lower risk of heart attack among fast metabolizers.

So, depending on your genes, caffeine could be both protective and detrimental to your heart health.

Other beneficial effects of caffeine include transient improvement of cognitive function, physical performance, and alertness.

However, different studies have produced inconclusive data about the potential protective effects of caffeine against certain diseases like Parkinson's and Alzheimer's. It is possible that the inconclusive results of these studies are due to the lack of genetic testing of caffeine metabolism in the subjects in these studies.

Based on the above, you may think that being a "slow metabolizer" may predispose you to skin conditions caused by caffeine.

Actually, you do not have to be a slow caffeine metabolizer to experience caffeine-induced skin conditions. While the rate at which your body metabolizes caffeine can influence the severity and duration of its effects, both slow and fast caffeine metabolizers can experience skin issues related to caffeine consumption.

Skin Diseases and Caffeine

There are a few mechanisms that are unique to caffeine's effect on the skin:

Vasodilation and Vasoconstriction

Caffeine has a dual role, as it may cause both vasodilation and vasoconstriction. As mentioned earlier, vasodilation is the dilation and widening of blood vessels, which is an indirect effect of caffeine on some blood vessels, including the facial ones. Caffeine stimulates blood pressure, which may manifest as increased blood flow to the face. That leads to exacerbation of rosacea.

Vasoconstriction is the narrowing of blood vessels, and it occurs because caffeine is a stimulant that blocks the action of adenosine, a neurotransmitter that promotes relaxation and dilates blood vessels. By blocking adenosine, caffeine leads to the constriction of blood vessels, which can temporarily reduce blood flow. This is why it is often used to alleviate headaches, as it can reduce the swelling of blood vessels that contribute to pain. After caffeine intake, vasoconstriction occurs first, followed by rebound vasodilation as the caffeine effect wears off.

Vasoconstriction can also lead to the narrowing of blood vessels, which can reduce blood flow to certain areas, including the delicate skin under the eyes. When blood flow is restricted, the blood vessels can appear darker or more pronounced through the thin skin, contributing to the appearance of dark circles under the eyes.

Dehydration

Caffeine is a diuretic that can lead to dehydration, which may cause dry, flaky skin. It also impairs the skin's barrier function, making it more susceptible to irritation and inflammation.

Sleep Disruption

Caffeine sensitivity can lead to sleep disturbances or insomnia. Poor sleep affects skin repair and regeneration, increasing the likelihood of skin issues.

Here is a summary of the mechanism of caffeine's impact on our skin.

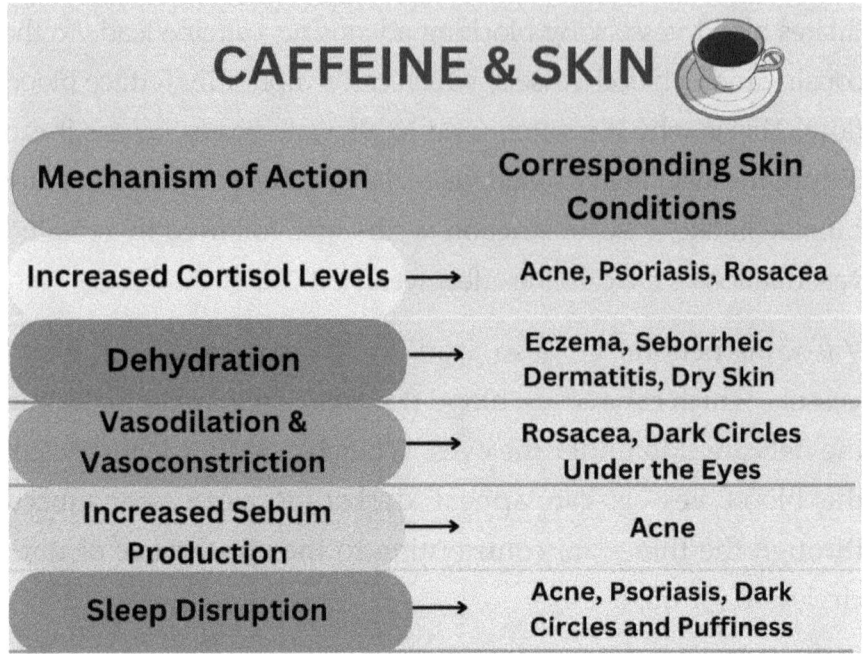

Figure 12.1 Mechanisms through which caffeine may affect the skin.

Managing Caffeine Sensitivity

The recommended daily dose of caffeine for "slow metabolizers" is 100-200 mg, with a lower dosage preferable.

In general, consuming more than 400 mg is not recommended, even for "fast metabolizers."

Obvious Sources of Caffeine:

Coffee: One of the most popular sources, with an average small cup (8 ounces) containing about 95 mg of caffeine.

Tea:

- ❖ Black Tea: 40-70 mg of caffeine per 8-ounce cup.
- ❖ Green Tea: 20-45 mg of caffeine per 8-ounce cup.

The amount of caffeine in tea depends on the type of leaves, the brewing time (longer brewing equals higher caffeine content), the number of tea leaves, and the water temperature (hotter water extracts more caffeine).

A few words about decaffeinated drinks:

Decaffeinated coffee and tea still contain small amounts of caffeine. For individuals with extreme caffeine sensitivity, even decaf can sometimes trigger symptoms.

Hidden Sources of Caffeine:

Content of Caffeine in Chocolate (per 1 ounce):

- ❖ Milk Chocolate: 5-10 mg.
- ❖ White Chocolate less than 1 mg
- ❖ Dark Chocolate 20-40 mg
- ❖ Soft Drinks contain, on average, 34 mg of caffeine per can.
- ❖ Energy Drinks: These can contain significant amounts of caffeine, with energy drinks typically having higher levels than soft drinks. The 8.4-ounce can may contain 80 mg, while certain energy shots may contain 200 mg of caffeine in a mere 2 ounces.

My recommendations are the same for soda and energy drinks: just say NO!

Caffeine-Containing Medications

Caffeine is a common ingredient in various medications, primarily due to its stimulant properties and its ability to enhance the effectiveness of certain drugs. Here are some types of medications that often contain caffeine:

Pain Relievers

- *Excedrin:* A combination of acetaminophen, aspirin, and caffeine, commonly used to treat headaches and migraines.
- *Midol Complete:* Includes acetaminophen, caffeine, and pyrilamine, which are used for menstrual cramps and related symptoms.

Medications for Fatigue

- *Vivarin, No Doz:* Over-the-counter caffeine tablets that are used to increase alertness and reduce fatigue.

Prescription Medications

- *Fioricet:* Contains butalbital, acetaminophen, and caffeine, prescribed for tension headaches.
- *Fiorinal:* Includes butalbital, aspirin, and caffeine, which are used for tension headaches.

Interestingly, several medications containing caffeine have been taken off the market in the last few years.

CHAPTER 14

Wine Sensitivity and Skin Conditions

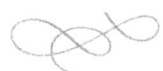

Wine contains several substances that may elicit skin reactions: histamines, sulfites, tannins and flavonoids, and alcohol.

Components of Wine: Histamines

We first learned about histamine in Chapter 4. *Histamine and Food Sensitivities*.

Let's review:

There are two sources of histamine available to you: histamine that you make in your body and histamine that you get from certain foods.

Your natural histamine is produced from an amino acid called histidine.

Histamine plays key roles in immune response, helps regulate stomach acid, and acts as a neurotransmitter.

Wine and fermented foods are examples of food sources of histamine, which is produced by lactic acid bacteria during fermentation and originates from histidine.

Components of Wine: Sulfites

Sulfites in wine are used primarily as preservatives to prevent spoilage and oxidation, helping to maintain the wine's freshness and stability. They have antimicrobial properties that inhibit the growth of unwanted bacteria and yeast, and they also act as antioxidants to prevent the wine from turning brown and developing off-flavors.

Sulfites occur naturally in small amounts during the fermentation process, but winemakers often add additional sulfites to ensure the wine's quality and longevity. Organic wines often have lower levels of added sulfites.

Some people are sensitive to sulfites and may experience allergic reactions or asthma-like symptoms after consuming wine with higher sulfite levels.

Components of Wine: Tannins and Flavonoids

Tannins, found in grape skins, seeds, and stems, can contribute to wine sensitivity. They are responsible for wine's astringent taste and can trigger migraines and other symptoms in sensitive individuals.

Flavonoids are anti-inflammatory compounds found in grapes and other plants. They provide red and purple hues to red wine. Flavonoids have been found to protect against heart disease.

So, tannins provide structure and aging potential, while flavonoids contribute to the sensory characteristics and potential health benefits of wine.

Components of Wine: Alcohol

Alcohol in wine, as well as alcohol in general, is detrimental to skin health by causing a variety of problems:

- *Vasodilation*: Alcohol dilates blood vessels, leading to redness and puffiness, contributing to or exacerbating rosacea.
- *Dehydration*: Alcohol is a diuretic. Dehydrated skin can become dry, flaky, and more prone to fine lines and wrinkles.
- *Inflammation:* Alcohol can cause inflammation in the body, which may exacerbate skin conditions like rosacea, eczema, and psoriasis. It can also lead to redness and puffiness in the skin.
- *Free Radicals:* Alcohol consumption can increase the production of free radicals, which are unstable molecules that can damage skin cells and accelerate aging.
- *Nutrient Depletion:* Excessive alcohol intake can deplete the body of essential nutrients like vitamins A, C, and E, which are important for maintaining healthy skin.
- *Poor Sleep:* Alcohol disrupts melatonin production, which regulates sleep. As we all know, lack of sleep results in dull skin, dark circles under the eyes, and a tired look.

Alcohol and Hormones

Alcohol consumption can raise cortisol levels, which can lead to a decrease in skin elasticity and early aging by breaking down collagen.

Alcohol can disrupt estrogen balance through several mechanisms. It increases the activity of the enzyme aromatase, which converts androgens into estrogens, leading to higher estrogen levels.

Chronic alcohol consumption also impairs liver function, reducing the liver's ability to metabolize and clear estrogen, resulting in its accumulation in the body.

Alcohol-induced weight gain, particularly in adipose tissue, further contributes to elevated estrogen levels, as fat tissue is a significant site of estrogen production.

Moreover, alcohol can disrupt the gut microbiome, affecting the reabsorption and metabolism of estrogen, which can exacerbate hormonal imbalances.

These combined effects can lead to an excess of estrogen, increasing the risk of various estrogen-related skin issues, such as acne and rosacea.

Alcohol can lead to increased insulin levels, which promote sebum production and clogged pores.

Alcohol Content in Wine

The alcohol content in wine varies widely, typically ranging from about 5% to 16% alcohol by volume (ABV). The specific alcohol content depends on factors like grape variety, region, climate, and winemaking techniques. Here are some averages:

- ❖ *Low-alcohol wines:* These often include sparkling wines and certain sweet wines, typically ranging from 5% to 11% ABV.
- ❖ *Standard table wines:* Most white and red wines fall in the range of 11% to 14% ABV.
- ❖ *High-alcohol wines:* Some red wines, fortified wines like Port and Sherry, and certain other wines can have an alcohol content ranging from 14% to 20% ABV or even higher.

Skin Diseases And Wine

Redness and flushing are among the most common skin issues linked to wine sensitivity, and this can be particularly pronounced with red wine.

Sulfites and tannins in wine can collectively increase the likelihood and severity of histamine-related symptoms, especially in individuals with histamine intolerance or sensitivity to these compounds. The sulfites might trigger histamine release, while tannins reduce the body's ability to break down histamine, leading to a higher concentration in the system and more pronounced symptoms.

Acne and Rosacea

Acne and rosacea are two common skin conditions that wine sensitivity exacerbates or triggers. Both conditions are characterized by a high inflammatory state, which wine can aggravate.

Other factors, such as histamine-induced vasodilation and alcohol-induced dehydration, may seal the deal.

Here is a summary of the mechanism of wine's impact on our skin.

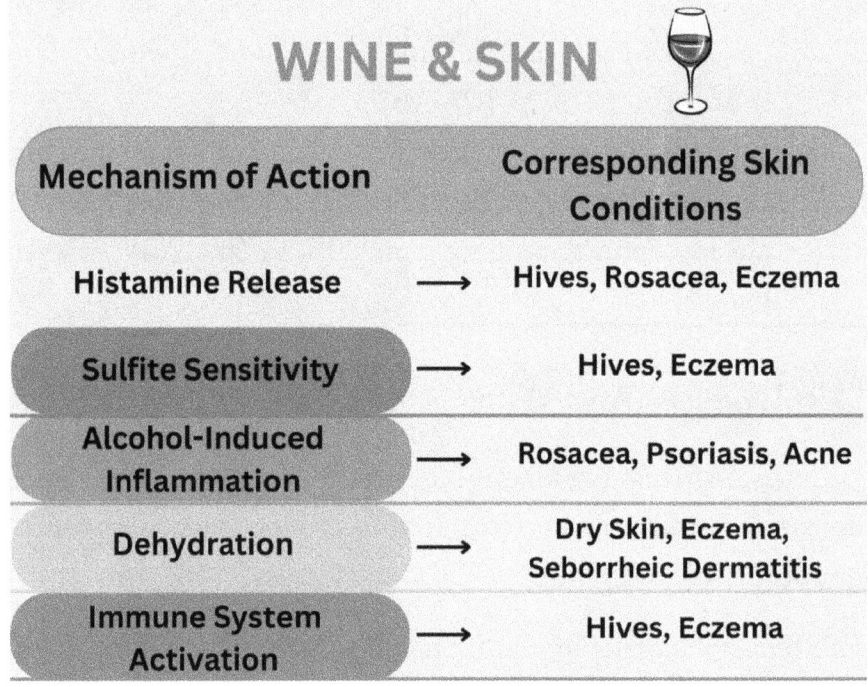

Figure 13.1 Mechanisms through which wine may affect the skin.

Managing Wine Sensitivity

Obvious Sources of Wine

❖ Wines: Red, white, rosé, sparkling wines, dessert wines, wine-based cocktails

Hidden Sources of Wine

❖ *Cooking Wines:* Wine is often used in cooking to enhance the flavor of sauces, soups, stews, and marinades. Dishes

like Coq au Vin, Beef Bourguignon, or certain pasta sauces may contain wine.
- ❖ *Vinegar:* Wine vinegar (both red and white) is made from fermented wine. It is often used in salad dressings, marinades, and sauces.
- ❖ *Sauces and Gravies* Pre-made sauces and gravies can sometimes contain wine as a flavor enhancer. This is especially common in gourmet or specialty products.
- ❖ *Desserts:* Some desserts, like certain cakes, tiramisu (Marsala wine), or fruit compotes, may contain wine or wine-based ingredients.
- ❖ *Condiments:* Some mustards, ketchup, and other condiments may use wine or wine vinegar as an ingredient.
- ❖ *Canned or Pre-Packaged Foods:* Some canned or pre-packaged foods, especially gourmet options, may include wine for flavoring, such as soups, pasta sauces, or stews.
- ❖ *Pickled Products:* Certain pickled vegetables or relishes might be prepared using wine vinegar.
- ❖ *Jellies and Jams:* Some jellies and jams, especially those labeled as gourmet or artisanal, may be made with wine or wine reductions for added flavor.

Sugar Content in Wine

Lastly, we should not forget that sugar is a significant component of many wines.

The sugar content in wine can vary significantly depending on the type and style of the wine.

- ❖ *Dry Wines:* These wines have little to no residual sugar left after fermentation. Most dry red and white wines fall into this category, typically containing less than 0-9 grams of sugar per liter.
- ❖ *Off-Dry Wines:* These wines have a slightly sweet taste due to a small amount of residual sugar. They generally contain between 10 and 18 grams of sugar per liter.
- ❖ *Sweet Wines:* These wines have a noticeable sweetness and higher sugar content, often due to stopping fermentation early or adding sugar. Sweet wines can contain more than 45 grams of sugar per liter. Examples include dessert wines like Sauternes, Port, and Moscato.
- ❖ *Sparkling Wines:* The sugar content in sparkling wines varies depending on the style, ranging from 3 to 50 grams per liter.

In summary, drinking wine in moderation and sticking with organic wines is the best way to get its benefits and avoid its dark side.

CHAPTER 15

Chocolate Sensitivity and Skin Conditions

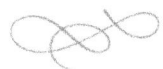

Let's break down the components of chocolate, a beloved treat for many of us.

Components of Chocolate

The core component of chocolate is cocoa, which includes cocoa solids and cocoa butter.

Cocoa contains several naturally occurring stimulants, such as theobromine, caffeine, and phenylethylamine. Since we already covered caffeine in *Chapter 12. Caffeine Sensitivity and Skin Conditions*, we will now focus on the other two components.

Theobromine is chemically similar to caffeine but has milder stimulant effects. It can still increase alertness and improve mood. Also, it is known to dilate blood vessels, which can lower blood pressure and improve blood flow. Like caffeine, theobromine has a diuretic effect.

Dark chocolate has higher concentrations of theobromine than milk chocolate due to its higher cocoa content.

Phenylethylamine (PEA) is also a stimulant. It is similar to amphetamines and functions as a neurotransmitter in the human brain. PEA is known for its potential mood-enhancing properties. It can promote the release of endorphins, inducing feelings of pleasure and well-being. This is why eating chocolate makes us feel happy. In some people, PEA might trigger migraines or headaches.

Other Components of Cocoa

- ❖ *Histamine:* Chocolate doesn't contain much histamine, but it tends to trigger our cells to release histamine.
- ❖ *Tyramine:* This naturally occurring monoamine is derived from the amino acid tyrosine. Tyramine can influence blood pressure by releasing norepinephrine, which can constrict blood vessels. Similar to phenylethylamine, it may trigger migraines in sensitive individuals. Individuals taking monoamine oxidase inhibitors (MAOIs) for depression or other conditions are often advised to avoid foods high in tyramine due to the risk of hypertensive crisis (a very high blood pressure). Thankfully, these antidepressants have largely been replaced by newer medications without these side effects.

Depending on the type of chocolate (milk, dark, white), there may be additional ingredients in chocolate:

- ❖ *Sugar*
- ❖ *Milk Solids* (present in milk chocolate)

- ❖ *Emulsifiers, such as Soy Lecithin* (used to maintain the texture and consistency of chocolate).
- ❖ *Flavorings and Preservatives* (Vanilla or other natural or artificial flavors may be added to enhance the taste of chocolate)
- ❖ *Nuts* (Many chocolates contain nuts or are processed in facilities that handle nuts)
- ❖ *Gluten* (Some chocolates may contain wheat-based ingredients like malt, barley malt, or other gluten-containing fillers that enhance texture or just be cross-contaminated with gluten during processing).

On this list of chocolate ingredients, you may recognize the foods we already reviewed as triggers for food sensitivities, such as sugar, milk, soy, nuts, and gluten. Unfortunately, due to its many triggering ingredients, chocolate may cause a bouquet of sensitivity reactions.

Skin Diseases and Chocolate

Here is a summary of the mechanism of chocolate's impact on our skin.

// Chocolate Sensitivity and Skin Conditions

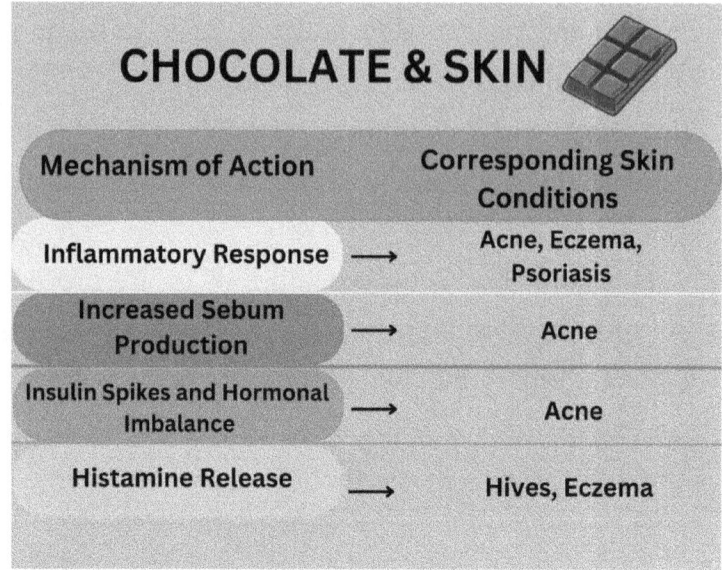

Figure 14.1 Mechanisms through which chocolate may affect the skin.

Managing Chocolate Sensitivity

Obvious Sources of Chocolate:

❖ Chocolate bars, truffles, chocolate cake, and hot chocolate

Hidden Sources of Chocolate:

❖ *Desserts:* Brownies, some cookies, and pastries
❖ *Snacks:* Some granola bars, trail mixes, and flavored nuts.
❖ *Beverages:* Chocolate-flavored coffee, milkshakes, and some energy drinks.

Chocolate-Free Alternatives:

❖ *Carob:* A naturally sweet alternative to chocolate, free from caffeine and lower in histamines.
❖ *Nut Butters:* Choose almond butter or sunflower seed butter unless you are sensitive to nuts and seeds!

CHAPTER 16

FODMAP Sensitivity and Skin Conditions

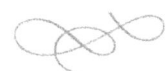

Definitions of FODMAPS

FODMAPs are a group of short-chain carbohydrates and sugar alcohols that are poorly metabolized in the small intestine of affected individuals.

FODMAPs stand for:

- ❖ *Fermentable:* These carbohydrates are fermented by gut bacteria, producing gas.
- ❖ *Oligosaccharides:* These include fructans (found in wheat, onions, and garlic) and galactans (found in legumes like beans and lentils).
- ❖ *Disaccharides:* This primarily refers to lactose, a sugar in dairy products like milk, yogurt, and soft cheese.
- ❖ *Monosaccharides:* This refers to fructose, a sugar in fruits, honey, and high-fructose corn syrup

❖ *Polyols:* These are sugar alcohols like sorbitol and mannitol found in some fruits and vegetables and artificial sweeteners.

Why FODMAPs May Cause Issues

Due to their chemical structure, these carbohydrates are not well absorbed in the small intestine, making it difficult for the lining to transport them efficiently into the bloodstream. When these poorly absorbed carbohydrates remain in the small intestine, they exert an osmotic effect, drawing water into the lumen of the intestine. This increased water content can lead to diarrhea and bloating.

Additionally, when FODMAPs pass through to the large intestine without being absorbed, they become a food source for the gut bacteria residing there. The bacteria ferment these carbohydrates, breaking them down into gases such as hydrogen, methane, and carbon dioxide. This fermentation process can produce significant amounts of gas, leading to symptoms such as bloating, flatulence, and abdominal pain. The combination of increased water and gas production can cause considerable discomfort and exacerbate symptoms in individuals with functional gastrointestinal disorders like irritable bowel syndrome (IBS) and SIBO (Small Intestinal Bacterial Overgrowth). Of note, in some literature, SIBO is considered a subtype of IBS.

How FODMAP Sensitivity is Diagnosed:

Hydrogen and methane breath tests are non-invasive diagnostic tools that can sometimes be used to identify specific FOD-

MAP intolerances, such as lactose or fructose malabsorption. These tests are designed to measure the amount of hydrogen and methane gases produced by the body after consuming a specific sugar solution. The presence and levels of these gases in the breath can provide valuable insights into how well the sugar is being absorbed in the small intestine.

Elevated hydrogen levels suggest the FODMAP being tested is being poorly absorbed. Unabsorbed carbohydrates are fermented by bacteria in the gut, leading to increased hydrogen production. Some people have gut bacteria that convert hydrogen into methane, leading to elevated levels of methane instead of hydrogen. Breath tests help identify which specific FODMAPs are not being absorbed properly.

Comprehensive stool tests are very helpful in identifying and quantifying the overgrowth of specific bacteria, making it helpful to diagnose SIBO. SIBO diagnosis may indirectly point to FODMAP sensitivity.

Skin Diseases and Fodmaps

Here is the summary of the mechanism of FODMAPs' impact on our skin.

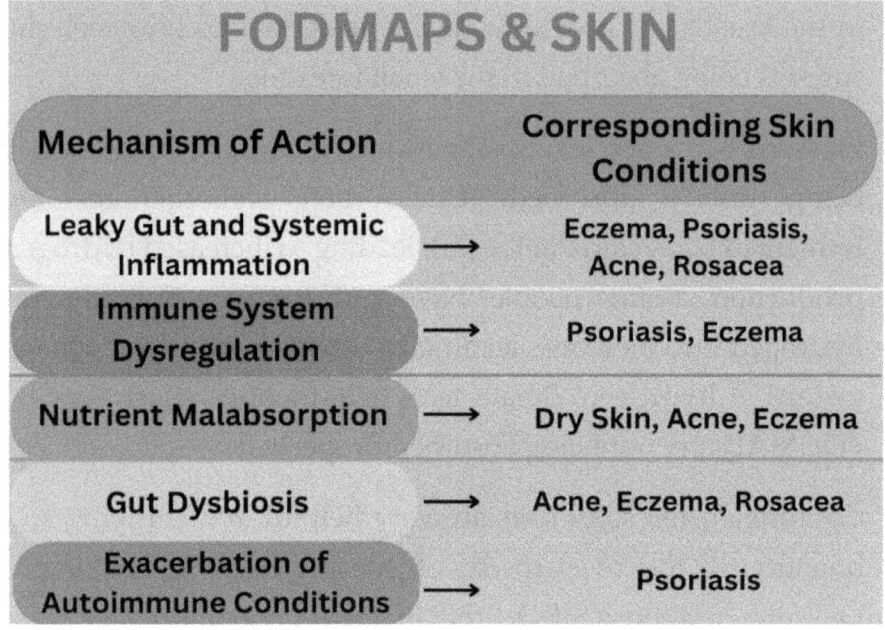

Figure 15.1 Mechanisms through which FODMAPs may affect the skin.

Managing FODMAP Sensitivity

Many foods in this group are very nutritious and cutting them out may be challenging.

Sources of FODMAPs:

Fermentable Oligosaccharides:

Fructans:

- ❖ Vegetables: Garlic, onions, leeks, asparagus, artichokes.
- ❖ Grains: Wheat, rye, barley

Galactans:

- ❖ Legumes: Lentils, chickpeas, kidney beans, black beans.

Disaccharides:

Lactose:

- ❖ Dairy Products: Milk, soft cheeses (e.g., ricotta, cream cheese), yogurt, ice cream.

Monosaccharides:

Fructose:

- ❖ Fruits: Apples, pears, mangoes, watermelon, cherries, sweetened drinks with high-fructose corn syrup.
- ❖ Sweeteners: Honey, high-fructose corn syrup, agave syrup.

Polyols:

Sorbitol:

- ❖ Fruits: Apples, pears, stone fruits (e.g., plums, apricots, cherries).
- ❖ Artificial Sweeteners: Sorbitol-containing sugar-free products (e.g., gum, candies).

Mannitol:

- ❖ Vegetables: Cauliflower, mushrooms, snow peas.
- ❖ Artificial Sweeteners: Mannitol-containing sugar-free products.

CHAPTER 17

Shellfish Sensitivity and Skin Conditions

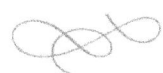

Components of Shellfish

Shellfish include a variety of marine animals, such as shrimp, crab, lobster, and mollusks like clams, oysters, and mussels. Here are the main components in shrimp and other shellfish that may trigger sensitivity and allergy:

Tropomyosin is the primary allergen found in the muscle tissue of shrimp and other shellfish. It can cause severe allergic reactions, including hives, swelling, difficulty breathing, and anaphylaxis.

Other allergens include arginine kinase, myosin light chain, hemocyanin (found in blood of shrimp) and paramyosin.

There is a known cross-reactivity between dust mites and shellfish. This cross-reactivity occurs because of the structural similarity between the proteins found in dust mites and those in shellfish, particularly tropomyosin, a protein that is a common allergen in both. This cross-reactivity is significant because individuals allergic to dust mites may also be at risk of developing an allergy to shellfish or vice versa.

Skin Diseases and Shellfish

Here is a summary of the mechanism of the impact of shellfish on our skin.

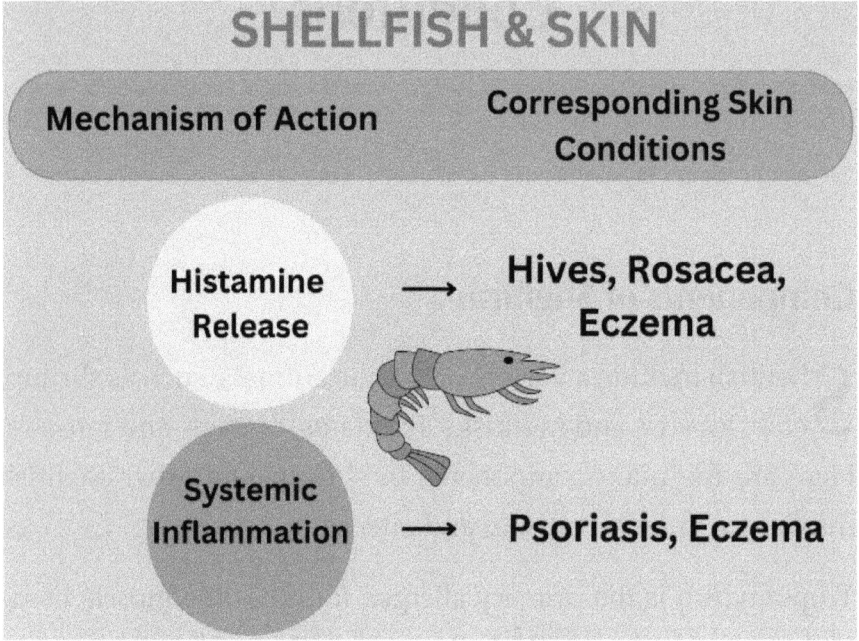

Figure 16.1 Mechanisms through which shellfish may affect the skin.

Interesting Fact

There used to be a notion in medicine that if you are allergic or sensitive to shellfish, you are allergic to the intravenous dye containing iodine used in CAT scans.

In fact, there is no cross-reactivity between shellfish and iodine. This misconception likely arises because shellfish allergies and reactions to iodine-based contrast dyes used in medical imaging are both common. However, the allergens in shellfish are specific proteins, not iodine. Therefore, an allergy to shellfish does not imply an allergy to iodine or iodine-based contrast dyes.

Managing Shellfish Sensitivity

Obvious Sources of Shellfish:

- ❖ *Seafood Platters:* These often contain a mix of shrimp, crab, lobster, clams, mussels, and oysters.
- ❖ *Sushi:* Many sushi rolls and sashimi include shellfish such as shrimp (ebi), crab (kani), and scallops.
- ❖ *Seafood Stews and Soups:* clam chowder, bouillabaisse, and gumbo
- ❖ *Pasta and Rice Dishes:* shrimp scampi, paella, and seafood risotto

Hidden Sources of Shellfish:

- ❖ *Imitation Crab Meat (Surimi):* Made from fish but flavored with crab extract, it can contain shellfish proteins.
- ❖ *Asian Cuisine:* Some broths and sauces used in Asian cooking, like fish sauce or oyster sauce, may contain shellfish.
- ❖ *Fried Foods:* Even if the food itself doesn't contain shellfish, it might be cooked in oil that has also been used for frying shrimp or other shellfish.
- ❖ *Supplements and Medications:* Some glucosamine supplements, often used for joint health, are derived

from shellfish shells. Use shellfish-free glucosamine supplements instead.

Shellfish Substitutes:

- ❖ *Non-shellfish Fish:* Use fish, such as cod, salmon, haddock, or tilapia, in place of shellfish in recipes.
- ❖ *Plant-Based Seafood:* These products are usually made from soy, legumes, seaweed, or other plant-based components. However, if they are processed in facilities that also handle shellfish, cross-contamination with shellfish may occur, so checking for allergen warnings is advised.

CHAPTER 18

Nightshade Vegetables Sensitivity and Skin Conditions

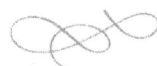

Common nightshade vegetables include tomatoes (technically fruits), potatoes (white and red), eggplants, and peppers (bell peppers, chili peppers).

Components of Nightshades

Nightshade vegetables contain several components that can cause food sensitivities in some individuals. The three main components are alkaloids, lectins, and saponins.

Types of Alkaloids:

❖ *Solanine:* Found in potatoes, particularly in the skins. While solanine is heat-stable and not destroyed by cooking, the concentration can be reduced by discarding the cooking water of boiled potatoes. Solanine can cause

digestive issues and neurological symptoms in sensitive individuals.
- ❖ **Tomatine:** As the name suggests, it is present in tomatoes, especially in unripe green tomatoes. It can cause gastrointestinal discomfort.
- ❖ **Capsaicin:** Found in peppers, capsaicin is responsible for the spiciness and can irritate the digestive tract. Interestingly, capsaicin has many health benefits. It is used as a topical analgesic for arthritic pain and muscle strains. It has also been implicated in weight loss, as it can increase metabolic rate. Additionally, it helps lower blood pressure.
- ❖ **Nicotine:** Present in very small amounts in some nightshades like tomatoes and eggplants.

Lectins

Lectins are proteins in nightshades that can bind to carbohydrates. They are also present in legumes, grains, milk, fruits, nuts, and seeds. Lectins may affect the digestive system by binding to the gut lining, causing gut irritation and nutrient malabsorption.

Saponins

Saponins are another group of compounds found in nightshade vegetables. They have soap-like properties, meaning they can form soap-like foams when mixed with water. Like lectins, saponins can disrupt gastrointestinal cell membranes, leading to a leaky gut.

Skin Diseases and Nightshades

Here is a summary of the mechanism of nightshades' impact on our skin.

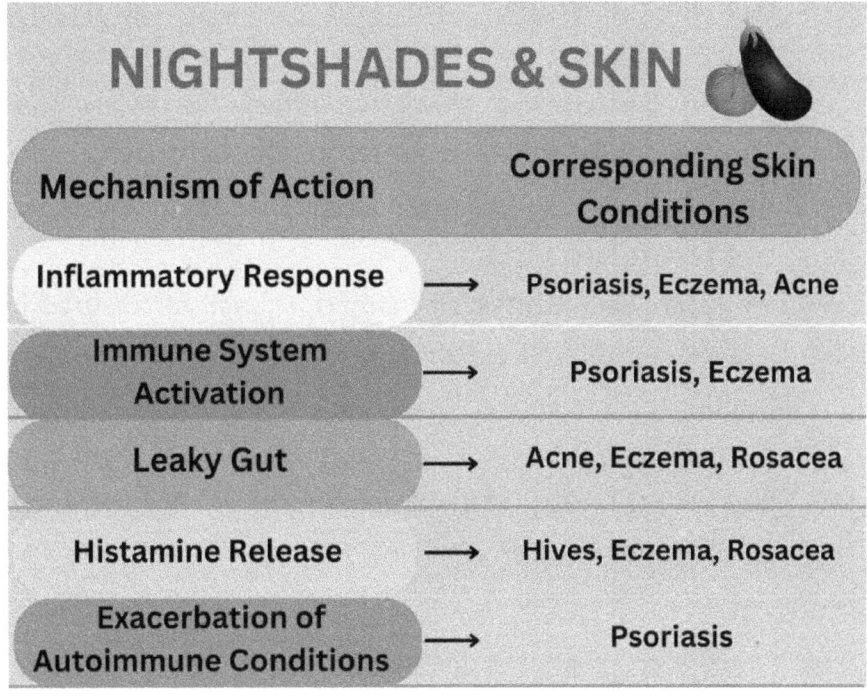

Figure 17.1 Mechanisms through which nightshades may affect the skin.

Managing Nightshade Sensitivity

Obvious Sources of Nightshades:

- ❖ Tomatoes, potatoes, eggplants, peppers

Hidden Sources of Nightshades:

- ❖ **Spices**: Paprika, chili powder, and cayenne pepper
- ❖ **Processed Foods**: Tomato paste, sauces, and soups
- ❖ **Condiments**: Ketchup, salsa, and hot sauce

- ❖ **Prepared Foods**: Some pre-packaged meals and snacks may include nightshade ingredients as flavor enhancers.

Alternatives to Nightshades:

- ❖ **Tomato Substitutes**: Use roasted beets or carrots as a base for sauces.
- ❖ **Potato Substitutes**: Sweet potatoes, parsnips, and turnips can be excellent replacements in many recipes. Cauliflower can be used to make mashed "potatoes" or even cauliflower fries.
- ❖ **Eggplant Substitutes**: Zucchini or squash can be used in place of eggplant in most dishes. Mushrooms can offer a similar texture and savory flavor.
- ❖ **Pepper Substitutes**: Use herbs like basil, thyme, or oregano to add flavor without the heat. For spice, try black pepper or ginger.

PART IV
Identifying Food Sensitivities

Now that we have discussed various foods and how and why they can trigger skin reactions, let's proceed with the ways to diagnose food sensitivities.

During patient consultations in our clinic, I often hear patients try to make connections between their skin issues and certain foods. It is always very valuable for me, as a clinician, as it indicates that that patient is tuned in to their body and that the patient is being proactive in their quest for health.

In our clinic, we recommend a food diary, an elimination diet, and food sensitivity testing.

Ideally, all three components should be implemented to get the best answer.

CHAPTER 19

Food Diary

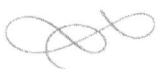

The idea of a food diary for food sensitivities is to document everything you eat for 4-6 weeks and your skin symptoms during the same period. You can assess your skin condition on a scale from 1 to 10 in terms of severity.

You can start a food diary by yourself now. You may then discover very interesting things about your health, and not only about your skin. You may discover how some foods deplete you, how some foods make you more focused, and much more.

When it comes to food sensitivities, it is both obvious and incredible that we are most sensitive to the foods that we eat habitually, day after day. It makes sense, but it also makes cutting out these trigger foods so difficult, as they feel like such a comfortable part of our routine!

Our clinic reviews patient food diaries and utilizes their results by incorporating them into testing and treatment plans. If there is an obvious connection, such as eating a chocolate bar and developing an acne flare-up several hours later, on more than one occasion, then our recommendation would be to eliminate chocolate in all forms for at least 3-6 weeks and then start slowly introducing it. However, if there are no clear correlations between any foods and flare-ups or the persistence of skin conditions, then a formal elimination diet would be the next recommended step.

CHAPTER 20

Elimination Diet

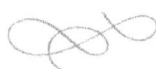

At our clinic, we implement what we call a "short-list" elimination diet (elimination of a few trigger food groups) and a "long-list" or traditional elimination diet (elimination of all trigger food groups).

As a physician, I favor a traditional "long-list" elimination diet, as it is more comprehensive and provides much more information. However, due to its restrictive nature, not every patient is willing to follow it. So, a short-list elimination diet is a compromise.

A "short-list" elimination diet is based on the elimination of 1-4 foods that are suspected of causing symptoms in a particular patient. If the food diary hints at gluten and milk sensitivity, then our short-food elimination diet will eliminate gluten and milk. For this "short-list" elimination diet to be the most productive, it should be followed for 4 to 6 weeks. Since it is based on the elimination of only a few foods, I find it much easier for patients to follow it.

However, we don't always have specific food suspects when evaluating food sensitivities, and in some cases, a food diary may be confusing because the patient may have multiple food sensitivities. Additionally, in cases of chronic or life-long skin conditions, such as persistent eczema, the food diary may not be as helpful, as the condition may look the same during the entire 4-6 weeks of food-diary documentation.

In that case, we recommend a "long-list" traditional elimination diet.

Phases of Elimination Diet

An elimination diet, whether "short-list" or "long-list," has three phases: elimination, reintroduction, and maintenance.

Let's look at the TRADITIONAL ELIMINATION DIET algorithm.

But first, before going on an elimination diet, please discuss it with your clinician!

Elimination Phase

- ❖ **Duration:** Typically lasts 3-6 weeks.
- ❖ **Process**: Food Groups to be eliminated: dairy, gluten, soy, eggs, nuts, shellfish, chocolate, processed foods, and artificial additives. Depending on the suspicion of additional food sensitivities for each patient, this phase could be further personalized, and more foods could be temporarily eliminated.

- **Purpose**: This phase allows the body to reset and get rid of the circulating IgG antibodies to potential trigger foods. We have discussed earlier that the half-life of IgG antibodies is 23 days. Based on that, the elimination phase should be at least 3 weeks. The goal is to observe if our skin symptoms improve once the IgG antibodies to potentially trigger foods are completely gone.

Reintroduction Phase

- **Duration**: Gradual process, usually taking several weeks.
- **Process**: In this phase, you reintroduce one eliminated food at a time every 3-5 days, monitoring for recurrence or worsening of skin symptoms. It is better to reintroduce one single food rather than a single food group. If symptoms occur, the food is removed again, and the process continues with other foods.
- **Purpose**: This phase identifies specific foods that trigger symptoms. This is the "aha" component of this diet, in which your body's symptoms point to the food culprit.

Maintenance Phase

- **Duration**: Several months to decades to rest of your life
- **Process**: This is a long-term eating plan that avoids or limits identified trigger foods while maintaining a balanced and nutritious diet.
- **Purpose:** Improve overall health, including specific skin conditions connected to ingestion of trigger foods.

The Negatives of Elimination Diet

I can't stress it enough: when it comes to the elimination diet, you need to be supervised by your clinician or nutritionist before, during, and after, as you will need medical and emotional support throughout this journey.

Nutritional Deficiencies

Eliminating multiple food groups can lead to the following nutritional deficiencies if not carefully managed: Calcium, vitamin D, vitamin B12, iron, fiber, protein, folate, and magnesium. Along the same lines, longer elimination diets may lead to hair loss, which may be devastating for many. Supplemental support is needed to prevent that.

Gastrointestinal Symptoms

Occasionally, diarrhea, constipation, bloating, gassiness, and even abdominal cramps may develop while on this diet. Sometimes, it is our body getting used to a new way of eating. Yet, sometimes, our body screams for certain vitamins and nutrients. That is why it is very important to be supervised by a clinician.

Overdoing It

Prolonged elimination of multiple food groups without proper planning can lead to overrestriction. In some cases, it may lead to a diet with elements of both fasting and elimination where each component is great on its own, but together, they can weaken the human body.

Erroneous Conclusions / Misidentification

Mistakes made during reintroduction, such as reintroducing foods too quickly or eating multiple foods of the same group, may lead to erroneous results. Another common mistake is eating large quantities of reintroduced foods. Even the healthiest food may trigger symptoms when not consumed in moderation.

Psychological Issues

The strict nature of an elimination diet can cause stress and anxiety around food choices and social eating situations. This can lead to an unhealthy relationship with food.

A few words about patients with eating disorders: I don't think it is a good idea to offer a traditional elimination diet to this vulnerable group of patients. It is more appropriate to do a "short-list" elimination diet of 1-2 foods, as a traditional elimination diet can trigger and exacerbate eating disorders, causing these patients more harm.

Challenges of Meal Preparation

Preparing meals can become more time-consuming and complex as you may need to find suitable substitutes for common ingredients and ensure all foods are free from the eliminated substances.

Social Awkwardness

Following such a strict diet may lead to social isolation and awkwardness. I recommend avoiding unnecessary explanations and focusing on your food choices. As an adult, you don't owe anybody any extensive explanations or disclaimers about what you eat!

In summary, only undertake an elimination diet under the supervision of a healthcare provider, especially if there are existing health conditions.

CHAPTER 21

Testing for Food Sensitivities

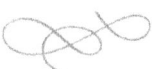

Food sensitivity tests are gaining increasing approval and usage among functional and traditional medicine providers. They should be used along with food diaries or elimination diets to help with diagnosis.

However, an elimination diet may not be for everyone, perhaps due to a history of an eating disorder or due to its restrictive nature, depending on the patient.

This is where food sensitivity testing comes in.

We mentioned earlier that food sensitivities are not stagnant; they may get worse, get better, or resolve with time. They are different from food allergies that do not change in adults.

This potentially transient nature of food sensitivities is because food sensitivities are often derivatives of other factors, such as leaky gut, infections, stress, etc.

When these root causes are addressed, food sensitivities can become milder or disappear.

Switching to a healthier lifestyle, including diet, supplements, exercise, and stress management, may reduce your food sensitivities. Nothing in our body functions alone: everything is interconnected!

Food sensitivity tests are gaining increasing approval and usage among functional and traditional medicine providers. They should be used along with food diaries or elimination diets to help with diagnosis.

However, an elimination diet may not be for everyone, perhaps due to a history of an eating disorder or due to its restrictive nature, depending on the patient.

This is where food sensitivity testing comes in.

We mentioned earlier that food sensitivities are not stagnant; they may get worse, get better, or resolve with time. They are different from food allergies that do not change in adults.

This potentially transient nature of food sensitivities is because food sensitivities are often derivatives of other factors, such as leaky gut, infections, stress, etc.

When these root causes are addressed, food sensitivities can become milder or disappear.

Switching to a healthier lifestyle, including diet, supplements, exercise, and stress management, may reduce your food sensitivities. Nothing in our body functions alone: everything is interconnected!

2 Types of Food Sensitivity Tests

Broadly speaking, food sensitivity tests are divided into IgG-based tests and non-IgG-based tests. IgG tests measure IgG and sometimes IgA antibodies in response to specific foods, indicating past exposure and potential immune reactions.

On the other hand, non-IgG-based tests assess food sensitivities using alternative biological markers. These may include changes in the size, volume, structure, or shape of white blood cells in response to food antigens. Some tests, like the Mediator Release Test (MRT) and ALCAT, focus on immune cell reactivity, while others, like electrodermal testing and applied kinesiology, rely on bioenergetic or muscle response assessments.

Let's take a closer look at each group and how they differ in their approach to identifying food sensitivities.

IgG-Based Food Sensitivities Testing

One of the most widely utilized methods for assessing food sensitivities involves measuring Immunoglobulin G (IgG) and/or Immunoglobulin A (IgA) antibodies in response to specific foods. Some of these tests require serum blood via a blood draw; others use a blood spot that involves a fingerstick. Of course, the fingerstick tests are more convenient, as they can be done at home.

IgG-based food sensitivity tests are designed to detect and quantify IgG antibodies against specific food antigens. What are antigens? Regarding food sensitivities, antigens are substances, usually proteins or molecules from foods, which trigger an immune response by stimulating the production of antibodies. The choice of method affects the accuracy, sensitivity, and clinical relevance of the results. Below are some of the commonly used techniques, but the list is incomplete, as new, and more sophisticated methods are being constantly developed.

Popular IgG Testing Techniques

Enzyme-Linked Immunosorbent Assay (ELISA)

ELISA is one of the most widely used techniques in IgG food sensitivity testing. It involves coating a microplate with food antigens and then adding a patient's serum to detect IgG antibodies that bind to these antigens. A secondary enzyme-linked antibody binds to IgG, producing a color change when a substrate is added. The intensity of the color correlates with the amount of IgG present. In short, ELISA is based on color change due to a chemical reaction. The intensity of the color is measured with a spectrophotometer. More intense color signifies more IgG antibodies and a higher reaction to a specific food.

Advantages:

- ❖ High sensitivity and specificity
- ❖ Relatively low cost
- ❖ Well-established methodology

Limitations:

- ❖ Variability in antigen preparation can affect accuracy.
- ❖ False positives may occur due to cross-reactivity.

Microarray-Based IgG Testing

This method also involves antigen-antibody interaction. Instead of the enzyme-linked reaction, like in ELISA, it uses imaging, such as fluorescence or chemiluminescence, to detect IgG binding to multiple food antigens simultaneously on a microarray chip. This test provides semi-quantitative results, ranking foods based on IgG response level.

Advantages:

- ❖ Allows testing of hundreds of foods at once
- ❖ Requires a very small blood sample
- ❖ More automation reduces human error

Limitations:

- ❖ Expensive compared to ELISA
- ❖ Limited availability in some labs

Multiplex Immunoassay (Bead-Based Technology)

This technique is somewhat like the Microarray technique, but instead of chips, it uses beads. A laser is used to detect fluorescent intensity that corresponds to the IgG response level for each food. Similarly to the Microarray technique, it can simultaneously detect multiple antigens.

Advantages:

- ❖ Higher precision and reproducibility than ELISA
- ❖ Faster turnaround time
- ❖ Capable of testing multiple antibody subclasses

Limitations:

- ❖ Requires sophisticated equipment and expertise
- ❖ Costlier than traditional ELISA

IgG Immune Complex Testing (Circulating Immune Complexes - CICs)

Instead of measuring free IgG antibodies, this test detects immune complexes formed between IgG and food antigens. These immune complexes are thought to contribute to systemic inflammation and chronic conditions.

Advantages:

- ❖ May offer more insight into inflammation than standard IgG tests
- ❖ Could better differentiate between harmless IgG responses and clinically significant reactions

Limitations:

- ❖ Less research backing compared to standard IgG testing
- ❖ Clinical relevance is still debated

IgG Subclass Testing

Instead of measuring total IgG, this method evaluates individual IgG subclasses (IgG1, IgG2, IgG3, IgG4). IgG4 is often the primary focus, as it is involved in immune tolerance and may not always indicate an adverse reaction. Some believe that elevated IgG4 may suggest adaptation rather than intolerance.

Advantages:

- ❖ May help differentiate between harmless exposure and problematic immune activation
- ❖ Could reduce overinterpretation of IgG results

Limitations:

- ❖ Clinical significance is not fully understood
- ❖ IgG4 presence does not necessarily correlate with symptoms

Clinical Considerations in IgG Testing

When it comes to IgG-based food sensitivity tests, the first challenge is interpretation of IgG tests. The IgG responses to foods are a normal part of our immune function and do not necessarily indicate food sensitivity in each case. Based on that, elevated IgG alone should not be the only criterion for eliminating foods; instead, results should be correlated with symptoms and confirmed with elimination diet and food reintroduction.

Another factor is variability between labs. Different labs use specific antigen preparations and that by itself may lead to inconsistencies, influencing test results.

Variability also stems from the usage of various combinations or types of IgG. Some tests measure total IgG, while others focus on IgG subclasses or immune complexes. That makes it difficult to accurately compare the results amongst different techniques.

To improve accuracy, many practitioners complement IgG testing with elimination diets and symptom tracking. In functional medicine, IgG testing is often integrated with other inflammatory markers, such as C-reactive protein (CRP) or zonulin, to assess gut permeability and systemic inflammation, providing a more comprehensive approach to food sensitivities.

IgG food sensitivity testing offers various methodologies, each with its strengths and limitations. ELISA remains the most used method due to its accessibility and cost-effectiveness, while newer technologies like microarrays and multiplex immunoassays enhance accuracy and efficiency. Microarray-based IgG Testing and Multiplex Immunoassay are more sensitive than ELISA, as they can detect very low levels of IgG antibodies, making it ideal for identifying even the weak immune responses to food antigens.

However, regardless of the testing method, IgG results should always be interpreted in the context of a patient's clinical presentation, symptoms, and dietary history to avoid unnecessary dietary restrictions and misdiagnosis.

Non-IgG Based Food Sensitivity Testing

Mediator Release Testing

The Mediator Release Test (MRT) offers a more comprehensive approach to food sensitivity testing by going beyond traditional antibody detection methods, such as IgG testing. Unlike tests that only measure immune antibody responses, the MRT assesses the release of inflammatory mediators—including histamines, prostaglandins, leukotrienes, and cytokines—from white blood cells when exposed to food antigens. As noted earlier, these mediators play a critical role in triggering systemic inflammation, which can manifest in various symptoms, including skin irritation, digestive disturbances, migraines, joint pain, and fatigue.

The MRT works by measuring changes in the size and volume of white blood cells following exposure to specific foods and additives. When a reactive food is encountered, immune cells release mediators, leading to cell shrinkage or swelling, which is detected through precise volumetric analysis. This method allows for a more functional assessment of how the immune system responds to different foods rather than relying solely on the presence of antibodies, which do not always correlate with clinical symptoms.

Advantages:

- ❖ MRT is more directly linked to inflammatory reactions that may cause symptoms.
- ❖ Can identify non-IgG-related food sensitivities (e.g., histamine or leukotriene-driven reactions)

Limitations:

- ❖ Does not identify the specific immune mediator (e.g., histamine vs. cytokines)

- ❖ More expensive and less widely validated than IgG testing
- ❖ Lacks standardization across different laboratories.

Lymphocyte Response Assay

The Lymphocyte Response Assay (LRA) is a specialized test designed to evaluate how white blood cells (namely, T lymphocytes) react to specific food antigens, chemicals, and environmental triggers, making it a powerful tool for identifying delayed hypersensitivity reactions. Unlike traditional antibody-based tests, such as IgG or IgE testing, which primarily detect past immune responses, the LRA provides real-time insights into the active state of the immune system, helping to uncover ongoing immune reactivity. By directly measuring how viable white blood cells respond when exposed to specific food and chemical antigens, the LRA can detect low-grade, persistent immune activation that may contribute to chronic inflammation.

During the test, a patient's lymphocytes are exposed to a panel of potential food and environmental triggers. The degree of immune cell activation is then assessed, allowing practitioners to identify which substances provoke a cellular inflammatory response.

Unlike IgG food sensitivity tests, which measure circulating antibodies that may not directly correlate with symptoms, the LRA assesses actual immune cell function and provides a more dynamic picture of current inflammatory responses. It helps distinguish between foods that merely produce an immune memory (IgG) and those that are actively causing systemic inflammation.

Advantages:

- ❖ Measures actual immune response: unlike IgG tests, LRA detects T-cell activation, identifying true delayed hypersensitivity reactions
- ❖ Comprehensive and functional—tests for foods, chemicals, molds, and environment triggers, making it useful for autoimmune and chronic inflammation cases

Limitations:

- ❖ Expensive and less available—costs more than IgG or MRT testing and requires specialized lab processing
- ❖ Results may vary—immune reactivity can fluctuate based on stress, infections, or medications, affecting test consistency.

Antigen Leukocyte Cellular Antibody Test

The ALCAT (Antigen Leukocyte Cellular Antibody Test) is a food sensitivity test that evaluates how the immune system reacts to various foods, chemicals, and environmental substances by measuring changes in white blood cell size and structure.

Certain foods or additives may cause immune cells to undergo morphological changes when exposed to potential triggers, indicating a sensitivity that could contribute to chronic inflammation and related symptoms.

Advantages:

- ❖ Measures white blood cell reactivity—detects immune cell changes in response to food and chemicals rather than just the presence of antibodies
- ❖ Covers a wide range of triggers and tests for foods, additives, molds, chemicals, and environmental substances
- ❖ Useful for inflammatory and digestive issues.

Limitations:

- ❖ Lacks standardization—results may vary between the tests.
- ❖ Scientific validation is limited compared to IgG or MRT testing.
- ❖ Does not identify specific immune pathways—measures overall cellular changes but does not pinpoint whether IgG, IgE, or T-cells are responsible for reactions.

Electrodermal Testing and Muscle Response Testing

Some alternative practitioners use non-invasive methods, such as electrodermal testing and applied kinesiology (muscle response testing), to assess food sensitivities.

Electrodermal testing measures changes in electrical conductivity when the body is exposed to different food frequencies. The patient typically holds a brass electrode or places their hand or finger on a sensor while the practitioner applies a probe to acupressure points, often on the fingers or palm. The probe is connected to a device that contains a sealed food extract. The device measures changes in skin resistance or conductivity. A drop in resistance is interpreted as sensitivity.

Muscle response testing evaluates muscle strength variations when encountering potential triggers. The patient holds a vial containing a food sample or places it under their tongue while the practitioner applies light pressure to a specific muscle, such as the arm. A noticeable muscle weakening is interpreted as a sign of food sensitivity, while maintained strength suggests tolerance.

Despite their use in holistic and alternative medicine, both methods lack standardized validation and are considered subjective and operator-dependent by conventional medical standards.

Advantages:
- ❖ Non-invasive and painless
- ❖ Immediate feedback (provides real-time responses based on muscle strength changes, which some practitioners use for personalized diet recommendations)

Limitations:

Lack of scientific validation—these methods are considered controversial in conventional medicine. There is no measurement of immune parameters pertinent to cells, immune system mediators, antibodies, or any targeted biochemical reaction directly correlating with a specific food.

Interpretation is subjective—results can vary depending on the practitioner's technique and patient expectations.

Lack of standardized protocols—different practitioners may use different testing approaches.

Comparison of Food Sensitivity Tests

The most accurate food sensitivity test depends on the purpose of testing, the specific immune response being assessed, and how results are interpreted. With an elimination diet being a gold standard, functional medicine providers typically combine clinical correlation with laboratory testing. Here is my breakdown of the most commonly used commercial tests and their accuracy:

1. *Elimination Diet with Reintroduction (Gold Standard)*
    - Accuracy: ★★★★★
    - **How it Works:** Involves removing suspected trigger foods for a period (usually 3–6 weeks), then systematically reintroducing them while tracking symptoms.
    - **Pros:** Identifies true symptomatic triggers, individualized, cost-effective, doesn't require a blood draw
    - **Cons:** Time-consuming, requires commitment and detailed tracking.

2. *Mediator Release Test (MRT)*
    - Accuracy: ★★★★☆
    - **How it Works:** Measures volumetric changes in white blood cells after exposure to food antigens, indicating the release of inflammatory mediators.
    - **Pros:** Assesses the functional immune response, not just antibodies; useful for systemic inflammation conditions.
    - **Cons:** Interpretation depends on clinical correlation, as it is not standardized. Some consider MRT unproven. Requires a blood draw.

3. *Lymphocyte Response Assay (LRA)*
   - **Accuracy:** ★★★★☆
   - **How it Works:** Evaluates lymphocyte reactivity to food and environmental antigens, identifying delayed hypersensitivity reactions (Type IV immune response) that may take hours or days to manifest.
   - **Pros:** Provides a direct measure of active immune cell responses; useful for detecting chronic inflammatory conditions such as autoimmune disorders, eczema, migraines, and gut permeability issues.
   - **Cons:** Requires specialized lab handling, and results must be interpreted in conjunction with symptoms for best accuracy. Requires a blood draw.

4. *Immunoglobulin G (IgG) Testing*
   - **Accuracy:** ★★★☆☆
   - **How it Works:** Detects IgG antibodies against foods, which may indicate immune memory rather than intolerance.
   - **Pros:** Provides a broad overview of food exposures, which is useful as a starting point. Can be done via fingerstick or a blood draw.
   - **Cons:** IgG presence alone does not confirm sensitivity; requires elimination diet confirmation.

4. *ALCAT Test*
   - **Accuracy:** ★★★☆☆
   - **How it Works:** Measures immune cell size changes in response to food antigens, similar to MRT but considered less precise.

- **Pros:** Identifies immune activation against foods.
- **Cons:** Higher variability between test results. Requires a blood draw.

To identify food sensitivities, the best approach is a combination of elimination diet, symptom tracking, and MRT or IgG testing. MRT tends to be the most functional test, as it assesses real-time immune reactivity rather than antibody presence alone. However, no test is perfect, so clinical symptoms should always be the deciding factor when making dietary changes.

Food Sensitivity Reports

Food sensitivity test results are typically presented in a graded format, categorizing foods into levels of reactivity (e.g., high, moderate, low, or no reaction). Many reports use a color-coded visual system with easy-to-read graphs or bars. Standard color designations are green for safe foods with no reactions, yellow for mild reactions, orange for moderate reactions, and red for severe reactions. The number of foods tested may range from 50-200, with the commonly tested food groups in food sensitivity tests including **dairy products, grains and gluten-containing foods, meats and poultry, seafood, eggs, nuts and seeds, legumes and beans, fruits, vegetables, oils and fats, spices and herbs, and beverages and additives.** Depending on the company and the specific test panel, each group may include 4 to 10 foods to assess individual immune reactivity.

Sample Food Sensitivity Report

FOOD GROUP	FOOD ITEM	SENSITIVITY LEVEL	VISUAL BAR
Grains	Wheat	Moderate	●●
	Oat	No Reaction	○
	Rice	No Reaction	○
	Barley	Mild	●
Nuts & Seeds	Peanuts	Mild	●
	Cashews	No Reaction	○
	Almonds	Severe	●●●
	Chia Seeds	No Reaction	○
Vegetables	Broccoli	No Reaction	○
	Onion	No Reaction	○
	Cauliflower	No Reaction	○
	Eggplants	Moderate	●●

Figure 21.1 Sample food sensitivity report

Interpreting Food Sensitivity Reports

When reviewing a food sensitivity report, it is essential to interpret the results in the context of symptoms and dietary habits rather than relying solely on the test outcome. Severe reactions typically indicate a high level of immune reactivity, suggesting that these foods may be major contributors to inflammation and symptoms. The best approach is to completely eliminate these foods for an extended period, usually 3 to 6 months, to allow the immune system and gut to heal. During this time, patients should monitor symptom resolution and consider additional functional medicine tests for gut health, inflammation, or intestinal permeability. After the elimination phase, a carefully controlled reintroduction can help determine if the food is truly problematic in the long term or if the immune response has subsided.

Moderate reactions suggest a lower but still significant immune response to the food, meaning it may not need to be permanently removed but should be limited or rotated in the diet. These foods can often be eliminated for a shorter period (4–8 weeks) and then reintroduced in a structured way, ideally under practitioner guidance. Mild reactions may indicate low-grade immune activation that might not cause noticeable symptoms unless consumed frequently or in large amounts. Rather than strict elimination, mild-reactive foods should be monitored and eaten in moderation, particularly in individuals with leaky gut, chronic inflammation, or autoimmune conditions. Ultimately, food sensitivity reports should be used as a guiding tool rather than a definitive diagnosis, with dietary changes tailored to the individual's symptoms, lifestyle, and overall health goals.

Retesting and Long-Term Management

Repeating a full food sensitivity panel is not usually necessary unless symptoms persist, or new concerns arise. However, re-evaluating gut health markers, such as intestinal permeability and microbiome balance, can provide valuable insights into long-term progress. In many cases, as gut health improves, food sensitivities become less severe or even disappear.

PART V

The Clear Skin Diet and Lifestyle Recommendations

CHAPTER 22

Clear Skin Diet

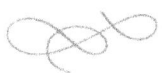

In a previous section, we reviewed foods known to cause sensitivities in some people. You may have noticed that most of the recommendations at the end of each chapter consisted of avoiding trigger foods.

This chapter is about adding food and supplements rather than taking them away!

The first thing about any food plan is addressing the root of healthy eating. As you have deduced from this book so far, a diet that is healthy for your gut is a diet that nourishes your whole body, including the skin.

You will see here some recommendations that are geared to skin health per se. However, no cell in our body exists on its own. All is connected.

Here is the Clear Skin Diet Summary

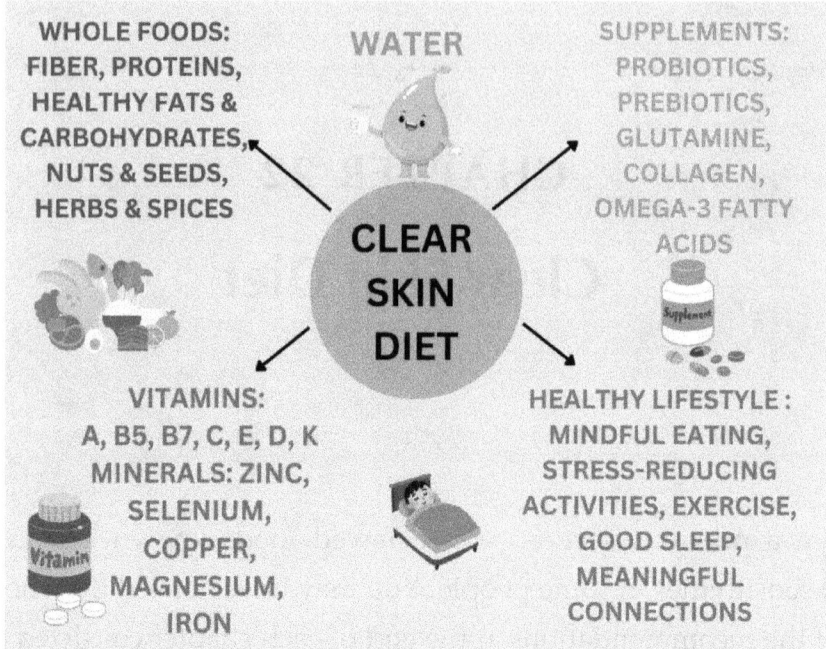

Figure 22.1 Clear Skin Diet template.

Meanwhile, let's unpack each element of the Clear Skin Diet one by one.

Whole Foods

Whole food is a natural food that is minimally processed and free from additives, preservatives, or artificial ingredients.

Here are the staples of a whole-food diet:

Fresh, Seasonal and Organic Fruits and Vegetables:

If you don't have access or can't afford organic fruit and vegetables, here are a few tips:

Rinse fruits and vegetables thoroughly under running water to remove surface residues from pesticides. Peel and trim the outer layers and peels of fruits and vegetables. It is unfortunate to have to do that, as many vitamins and nutrients are housed within these layers and peels. If possible, you may consider growing your own fruits and vegetables!

Whole Grains:

Whole grains are grains that contain all three parts of the grain kernel: the bran (outer layer), germ (the core), and endosperm (the middle layer). Each layer has specific nutrients:

- ❖ **Bran** contains fiber, antioxidants, and B vitamins.
- ❖ **Germ** has vitamins, minerals, healthy fats, and protein.
- ❖ **Endosperm** contains carbohydrates, some protein, and small amounts of vitamins and minerals.

Examples of Whole Grains:

- ❖ Brown rice, quinoa*, oats, whole wheat, barley, bulgur, farro, millet, spelt, dark rye, amaranth.
- ❖ Of note, quinoa is technically a seed. It is a complete protein with all nine essential amino acids. It is high in fiber and contains several vitamins and minerals.

Fiber

This is a good place to discuss the role of fiber in our diet:

Let's start with fiber as a component of whole food.

Fiber is a requirement of any healthy nutritional plan. Fiber is a type of carbohydrate that the body cannot digest. Unlike other carbohydrates that break down into sugar molecules, fiber passes through the digestive system relatively intact. There are two main types of dietary fiber: soluble and insoluble.

- *Soluble Fiber* dissolves in water to form a gel-like substance. It can help lower blood cholesterol and glucose levels. Soluble fiber is found in foods such as oats, barley, nuts, seeds, beans, lentils, peas, and some fruits and vegetables, like apples, pears, carrots, and sweet potatoes.
- *Insoluble Fiber* does not dissolve in water and adds bulk to the stool, helping food pass more quickly through the stomach and intestines. Insoluble fiber is found in foods such as wheat bran, brown rice, and vegetables like broccoli, green beans, cabbage, and spinach.

Many fruits and vegetables contain both soluble and insoluble fiber.

Why Fiber is Important

- *Digestive Health:* Fiber prevents constipation by adding bulk to the stool. It also supports a healthy gut microbiome by serving as food for beneficial bacteria.
- *Weight Management:* High-fiber foods are typically more filling, which can help control appetite and support weight loss or maintenance by promoting a sense of fullness.
- *Blood Sugar Control:* Soluble fiber, found in foods like oats and legumes, slows the absorption of sugar, which can help maintain steady blood sugar levels and reduce the risk of type 2 diabetes.

- ❖ *Heart Health*: Fiber can help lower cholesterol levels by binding to cholesterol particles and removing them from the body. This can reduce the risk of heart disease.
- ❖ *Colon Health*: A diet high in fiber can reduce the risk of developing colorectal cancer by promoting regular bowel movements and reducing the time harmful substances spend in the colon.
- ❖ *General Well-Being*: Fiber supports overall health by aiding in the absorption of nutrients and promoting a balanced diet.

Fiber Requirements

Here are the daily fiber intake recommendations according to the Dietary Guidelines for Americans based on age and gender.

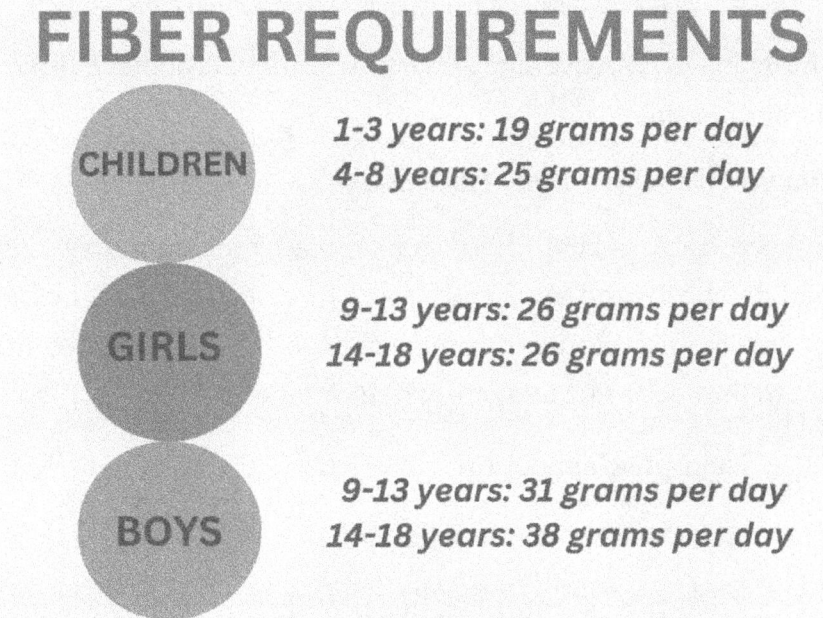

Figure 22.2 Fiber requirements in children

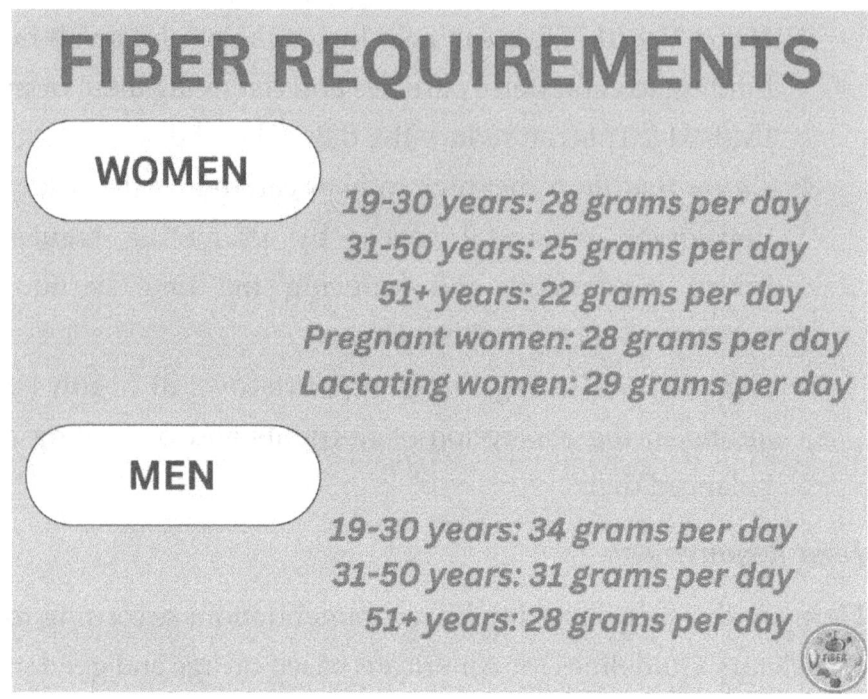

Figure 22.3 Fiber requirements in women and men.

Unfortunately, an average American adult eats about 15 grams of fiber per day.

How to Calculate a Daily Fiber Intake

To keep track of daily fiber intake, read nutrition labels, use food databases and apps and keep a food diary. This is how to sum up the fiber content from all the foods you consumed in a day to find out your total daily fiber intake.

Example Calculation

Suppose you ate the following in a day:

Breakfast: 1 cup of oatmeal (4 grams of fiber) with 1 banana (3 grams of fiber)

Lunch: A sandwich with 2 slices of whole wheat bread (4 grams of fiber each, total 8 grams) and 1 cup of cooked spinach (4 grams of fiber)

Snack: 1 apple (4 grams of fiber)

Dinner: 1 cup of cooked lentils (15 grams of fiber) with 1 cup of cooked broccoli (5 grams of fiber)

Total fiber intake for the day:
4 + 3 + 8 + 4 + 4 + 15 + 5 = 43 grams of fiber

Macronutrients: Carbohydrates

Carbohydrates are not our enemies. They are the body's main source of energy. By providing an adequate energy source, carbohydrates spare protein from being used as an energy source. This allows the protein to be used for its primary functions of building and repairing tissues. Glucose, the end product of carbohydrates' breakdown, is needed for brain function, physical endurance and strength, efficient fat burning, and more.

The recommended carbohydrate intake is **45-65% of your total daily calories**, ensuring you get enough energy and nutrients to support your body's functions. Limit intake of added (simple) sugars to less than 10% of total daily calories.

Macronutrients: Proteins

Protein is essential for your body because it helps build and repair tissues, including muscles, skin, and organs. It also makes enzymes and hormones that help your body function properly. Protein gives you energy and helps keep your immune system strong.

How Much Protein You Need

The amount of protein you need daily depends on age, sex, and activity level.

For most adults, the amount needed is 46 -56 grams of protein per day.

A simple rule of thumb is to get about 10-35% of your daily calories from protein.

To calculate your daily protein intake, use the following:

Sedentary Adult: 0.8 grams per kg

Moderately Active Adult: 1 to 1.5 grams per kg

Very Active Adult/Athlete: 1.2 to 2 grams per kg

Plant-Based Proteins

Legumes:

- *Lentils:* High in protein, fiber, iron, and folate.
- *Chickpeas:* Also known as garbanzo beans, they are versatile and rich in protein and fiber.
- *Black Beans:* Packed with protein, fiber, and various vitamins and minerals.
- *Kidney Beans:* High in protein, fiber, and iron.

Nuts and Seeds:

- *Almonds:* Provide protein, healthy fats, and vitamin E.
- *Chia Seeds:* Rich in protein, omega-3 fatty acids, and fiber.
- *Hemp Seeds:* Contain complete protein, healthy fats, and minerals.
- *Pumpkin Seeds:* High in protein, magnesium, and zinc.
- *Flaxseeds:* Provide protein, omega-3 fatty acids, and fiber.

Soy Products:

- *Tofu:* Made from soybeans, it's a versatile protein source.
- *Tempeh:* Fermented soy product that's high in protein and probiotics.
- *Edamame:* Young soybeans that are high in protein and fiber.

Whole Grains:

- *Quinoa:* A complete protein with all nine essential amino acids, plus fiber and minerals.
- *Farro:* An ancient grain high in protein, fiber, and various nutrients.
- *Amaranth*: Another complete protein grain rich in vitamins and minerals.

Plant-Based Protein Powders:

- *Pea Protein:* Derived from yellow split peas, it's high in protein and easily digestible.
- *Hemp Protein:* Made from hemp seeds, it's a good source of protein and healthy fats.
- *Brown Rice Protein:* A hypoallergenic option that's high in protein.

Vegetables:

- ❖ *Spinach:* Contains a moderate amount of protein and is rich in vitamins and minerals.
- ❖ *Broccoli:* High in protein compared to other vegetables, along with fiber and vitamins.
- ❖ *Brussels Sprouts:* Provide protein, fiber, and various nutrients.

Animal-Based Proteins

Lean Meats:

- ❖ *Chicken Breast:* High in protein, low in fat, and a good source of B vitamins and minerals.
- ❖ *Turkey:* Similar to chicken, turkey is lean and rich in protein and nutrients.
- ❖ *Lean Cuts of Beef:* Cuts like sirloin, tenderloin, and round are lower in fat and provide iron, zinc, and B vitamins.
- ❖ *Pork Tenderloin:* A lean cut that is high in protein and relatively low in fat.

Fish and Seafood:

- ❖ *Salmon:* Rich in omega-3 fatty acids, high-quality protein, and vitamins D and B12.
- ❖ *Tuna:* High in protein and omega-3 fatty acids, with low-fat content.
- ❖ *Cod:* A lean fish that is high in protein and low in fat.
- ❖ *Shrimp:* Low in fat and calories but high in protein and nutrients like selenium and vitamin B12.

Eggs:

- ❖ *Whole Eggs:* Provide high-quality protein, healthy fats, vitamins, and minerals like choline and vitamin D.
- ❖ *Egg Whites:* Almost pure protein, with no fat or cholesterol.

Dairy Products:

- ❖ *Greek Yogurt:* High in protein, probiotics, and calcium, with options available in low-fat or non-fat varieties.
- ❖ *Cottage Cheese:* A high-protein, low-fat dairy option rich in calcium and other nutrients.
- ❖ *Low-Fat Milk:* Provides protein, calcium, and vitamin D with lower fat content.

Other:

- ❖ *Game Meats:* These are venison and bison, which are typically leaner than conventional meats and are rich in protein and nutrients.

Macronutrients: Fats

Three types of fats are commonly found in our diet: saturated fats, monounsaturated and polyunsaturated fats, and trans fats.

Saturated, unsaturated, and trans fats differ significantly in their chemical structure, physical state, sources, and health impacts.

Saturated fats have no double bonds between the carbon atoms in their fatty acid chains, resulting in a straight structure that is typically solid at room temperature. Excessive intake of saturated fats can raise LDL (bad) cholesterol levels, increasing the risk of heart disease and stroke.

Unsaturated fats, including monounsaturated and polyunsaturated fats, have one or more double bonds in their carbon chains, creating kinks that prevent tight packing and are generally liquid at room temperature. These fats can help reduce LDL cholesterol levels and are beneficial for heart health, with omega-3 and omega-6 fatty acids playing essential roles in brain function and cell growth.

Trans fats, created through hydrogenation, have a straight, rigid structure due to the specificity of their double bonds, making them solid or semi-solid at room temperature. They are found in partially hydrogenated oils in many processed foods, such as margarine, shortening, fried foods, and baked goods. Trans fats raise LDL cholesterol levels and lower HDL (good) cholesterol levels, significantly increasing the risk of heart disease, stroke, and type 2 diabetes, leading many countries to regulate their use in the food supply.

Your total fat intake should be 20-35% of your total daily calories, and it should mostly include healthy monounsaturated and polyunsaturated fats.

Healthy Sources of Monounsaturated and Polyunsaturated Fats

- ❖ **Olive Oil** (cold-pressed or extra-virgin is better)
- ❖ **Avocados** (cold-pressed or extra-virgin is better)
- ❖ **Nuts**: Almonds, cashews, pecans, walnuts
- ❖ **Seeds**: Pumpkin seeds, sesame seeds, flaxseeds, chia seeds, hemp seeds, sunflower seeds

- ❖ **Nut Butters**: Almond butter, cashew butter.
- ❖ **Fatty Fish**: Salmon, mackerel, sardines, trout
- ❖ **Olives**
- ❖ **Tofu**

Saturated Fats

While saturated fats are mostly found in junk food (fast food, snacks, processed meats, baked supermarket food), some sources can be part of a healthy diet, particularly those found in whole, unprocessed foods. Examples of saturated fats to be used in moderation are grass-fed butter, full-fat dairy products, and dark chocolate.

Trans Fats

When it comes to trans fats, please avoid them completely.

Herbs and Spices

Herbs and spices are packed with vitamins, minerals, and antioxidants that help keep your body healthy by fighting off free radicals and reducing inflammation. Plus, they add fantastic flavor to your food without extra calories, salt, or unhealthy fats. Many herbs and spices have special health benefits, like anti-inflammatory, antimicrobial, and digestive support properties.

Fresh Herbs

- ❖ **Basil**: Rich in antioxidants, vitamins A, K, and C, and has anti-inflammatory properties.

- **Parsley**: High in vitamins A, C, and K, and supports bone health and digestion.
- **Cilantro (Coriander)**: Contains vitamins A, C, and K, and has detoxifying and digestive benefits.
- **Mint**: Helps with digestion, contains vitamins A and C, and has antioxidant properties.
- **Rosemary**: Contains antioxidants and anti-inflammatory compounds and supports memory and concentration.
- **Thyme**: Rich in vitamins C and A and has antimicrobial and respiratory benefits.
- **Oregano**: High in antioxidants, vitamins K and E, and has antimicrobial properties.
- **Sage**: Contains vitamins K and A and has anti-inflammatory and brain-boosting properties.
- **Dill**: Provides vitamins A and C and supports digestion and bone health.
- **Chives**: Rich in vitamins A and C and support immune health and digestion.
- **Tarragon**: Contains vitamins A and C and has digestive and anti-inflammatory benefits.
- **Lemongrass**: Rich in antioxidants, supports digestion, and has anti-inflammatory properties.

Nuts and Seeds

If you are sensitive to nuts or seeds, you may skip this section. However, for those without sensitivities, nuts and seeds are an important staple of a healthy diet.

A disclaimer: nuts and seeds should be eaten in moderation for several reasons:

They are very calorie-dense, meaning they contain many calories in a small serving. Overconsumption can lead to an excessive calorie intake, which may contribute to weight gain if not balanced with physical activity.

While nuts and seeds are a good source of healthy fats, consuming too much fat, even the healthy kind, can still contribute to a high-fat diet. This can affect the balance of other macronutrients (carbohydrates and proteins) in your diet.

It's easy to overeat nuts and seeds because they are small and often come in convenient snack forms. Practicing portion control helps ensure that you enjoy the health benefits without consuming too many calories.

Some nuts and seeds, such as sunflower seeds, are high in omega-6 fatty acids. While these are essential fats, excessive intake can disrupt the balance between omega-6 and omega-3 fatty acids, potentially leading to inflammation and other health issues.

Eating large quantities of nuts and seeds can cause digestive issues, such as bloating or gas, for some people.

Healthy Nuts

- ❖ **Almonds**: Rich in protein, healthy fats, fiber, vitamin E, and magnesium.
- ❖ **Walnuts**: High in omega-3 fatty acids, antioxidants, and several vitamins and minerals.

- **Cashews**: Provide healthy fats, protein, copper, magnesium, and vitamin K.
- **Pistachios**: Contain protein, fiber, antioxidants, and vitamins B6 and E.
- **Brazil Nuts**: Excellent source of selenium, healthy fats, and protein.
- **Hazelnuts**: Rich in healthy fats, vitamin E, fiber, and magnesium.
- **Macadamia Nuts**: High in monounsaturated fats, fiber, and several vitamins and minerals.
- **Pecans**: Contain healthy fats, fiber, antioxidants, and vitamin E.

Healthy Seeds

- **Chia Seeds**: High in omega-3 fatty acids, fiber, protein, and antioxidants.
- **Flaxseeds**: Rich in omega-3 fatty acids, fiber, lignans, and several vitamins and minerals.
- **Pumpkin Seeds**: Provide protein, healthy fats, magnesium, and antioxidants.
- **Sunflower Seeds**: Contain healthy fats, protein, vitamin E, and selenium.
- **Hemp Seeds**: Rich in omega-3 and omega-6 fatty acids, protein, and several vitamins and minerals.
- **Sesame Seeds**: High in healthy fats, protein, fiber, and several vitamins and minerals.
- **Poppy Seeds**: Provide healthy fats, fiber, protein, and several vitamins and minerals.

❖ **Quinoa:** Technically a seed, it is a complete protein with all nine essential amino acids, high in fiber and several vitamins and minerals.

Water

Water should be a key part of your diet for several important reasons that affect your overall health and well-being. Since 60% of your body is water, it is crucial to stay hydrated to keep all your bodily fluids in balance. Water is needed for digestion, absorption, circulation, making saliva, moving nutrients around, and preventing constipation by flushing out toxins from your body. When you sweat and breathe, water helps keep your body temperature in check, so you don't overheat.

Staying hydrated is key to maintaining your physical and cognitive performance. Without enough water, you might feel muscle fatigue, lose coordination, and have decreased strength and endurance. Drinking enough water helps you stay focused, alert, and sharp. Dehydration can mess with your mood and brain power.

It is no surprise that water keeps skin elastic and moist, reducing dryness and wrinkles.

Drinking enough water every day helps your body perform these vital functions efficiently. Aim for at least 8 cups (64 ounces) of water a day, but remember, your needs might vary based on your age, weight, activity level, and the climate you live in. A simple piece of advice: Don't forget to drink water when you are thirsty. Sometimes, thirst could be confused with hunger and may lead to overeating.

Vitamins and Minerals for Clear Skin

Is a Daily Multivitamin Necessary?

The necessity of a daily multivitamin can depend on various factors, including diet, health status, age, and lifestyle.

If you follow a well-balanced diet that includes a variety of fruits, vegetables, whole grains, protein, and healthy fats, you may not need a daily multivitamin. Nutrients are best absorbed from food sources.

There are several situations that preclude this from happening:

Limited access or lack of time to plan a healthy diet: It is not easy for an average person who is juggling work, family, and other commitments to follow a healthy diet. Time and planning are required to eat clean, organic food with no additives. Due to the difficulty in accessing healthy foods, we end up compromising by eating suboptimal foods: fast food, GMO-altered artificial food, strange snacks, etc. This makes one deficient in macronutrients, vitamins, and minerals.

Poor dietary habits, stress, toxins, and other factors can lead to a leaky gut and food sensitivities, which compromise our ability to absorb and extract vitamins and minerals from food.

Certain dietary habits, such as vegetarianism, veganism, calorie-restricted and intermittent fasting diets, might lack specific nutrients such as B12, iron, or omega-3 fatty acids, which could justify the use of multivitamins.

Getting older often diminishes our ability to absorb and extract nutrients from foods. Common age-related recommended micronutrients are vitamin D, vitamin B12, and magnesium.

Having medical diseases, undergoing intestinal surgery, or taking certain prescription medications may lead to mineral and vitamin deficiencies, necessitating supplementation.

Many of us fall into one of these categories, which is why the demand for multivitamins and supplements has increased significantly.

In line with this book's theme, we will focus on micronutrients that are beneficial for the skin. However, I recommend discussing the full range of vitamins and minerals your body needs with your healthcare provider. A personalized approach is the key to success.

Supplements For Clear Skin: Vitamins

Vitamin A

Vitamin A helps to stimulate the production of new skin cells, reduce fine lines and wrinkles, and improve skin texture.

Retinoids (topical derivatives of vitamin A) are effective in treating acne and reducing signs of aging.

Food sources of vitamin A include carrots, sweet potatoes, spinach, and other leafy greens, as well as animal products like liver and eggs.

Vitamin C

Vitamin C is a powerful antioxidant that helps protect the skin from free radical damage, supports collagen synthesis, and improves skin elasticity and brightness. Vitamin C is present in citrus fruits (oranges, lemons), strawberries, bell peppers, and broccoli.

Vitamin E

Vitamin E acts as an antioxidant, protecting skin cells from damage. It helps moisturize the skin and can aid in the healing of scars and burns. Vitamin E can also help reduce UV-induced skin damage. Nuts, seeds, spinach, and avocados are good sources of vitamin E.

Vitamin D

Vitamin D is essential for skin cell growth, repair, and metabolism. It can help prevent skin aging and has a therapeutic effect on psoriasis. In fact, calcipotriene, a topical medication commonly used for psoriasis, is a synthetic derivative of vitamin D. The food sources of vitamin D are sunlight exposure, fortified foods, fish, and dairy products.

Vitamin K

Vitamin K is important for healing wounds and reducing the appearance of scars, dark spots, and under-eye circles. Vitamin K can help improve skin elasticity and heal bruises and cuts more quickly. Food sources of vitamin K include leafy green vegetables, such as kale, spinach, and broccoli, as well as fish, meat, and eggs.

B Vitamins

- ❖ **Biotin (B7)** promotes healthy skin, hair, and nails.
- ❖ **Pantothenic Acid (B5)** hydrates skin and improves acne.

Sources of B vitamins include whole grains, meat, eggs, nuts, seeds, and legumes.

Supplements For Clear Skin: Minerals

Zinc

Zinc is essential for normal hair and nail growth and reduces inflammation in acne. Food sources of zinc include meat, shellfish, dairy products, nuts, seeds, and whole grains.

Selenium

Selenium protects skin from UV-induced damage. It is important for skin elasticity and reduces signs of aging. The food sources of selenium are Brazil nuts, seafood, eggs, and whole grains.

Copper

Copper is necessary for the production of collagen and elastin and helps in the formation of melanin, the pigment that gives skin its color. Shellfish, nuts, seeds, whole grains, and dark leafy greens are good sources of copper.

Magnesium

Magnesium reduces inflammation and promotes healing while improving skin hydration. It may also reduce the severity of acne. Food sources of magnesium include nuts, seeds, whole grains, and leafy green vegetables.

Iron

Iron is essential for oxygen transport to skin cells, supporting a healthy complexion and skin tone. Adequate iron levels are necessary to prevent pale skin and promote healthy cell function. The food sources of iron are red meat, poultry, seafood, beans, and leafy green vegetables.

Probiotics

The term "probiotic" comes from the Greek words "pro," meaning "for," and "biotic," meaning "life." Probiotics are often referred to as "good" bacteria. Probiotics have been used for thousands of years. Fermented foods like yogurt, sauerkraut, and kimchi were consumed for their health benefits long before the term "probiotics" was coined.

The role of probiotics has become more prominent as more research has come out about gut microbiome and leaky gut. Probiotics are now viewed as the "balancers" of the gut microbiome.

The gut immune system must protect against harmful bacteria and provide tolerance to microorganisms that are harmless. Probiotics play a significant role in helping the immune system accomplish this task.

As a clinician, I first heard about probiotics in the context of antibiotics years ago. As antibiotics wipe out both good and bad gut bacteria, that allows opportunistic fungus to take their place. That is why skin, oral, and vaginal fungal infections are seen in people who have been on frequent or prolonged course of antibiotics, especially the broad-spectrum ones, which kill many different species of bacteria.

Probiotics have been found to be helpful in weight loss by helping with metabolism through gut microbiome stabilization.

In terms of mental health, some studies suggest that probiotics may help reduce symptoms of anxiety and depression. Additionally, special probiotics formulas now aim to improve cognition.

In addition to helping balance the gut microbiome and mitigating leaky gut, probiotics have the following DIRECT effects on your skin through several mechanisms.

Here are some ways probiotics can positively influence the skin:

- ❖ Strengthen skin barrier and promote moisture retention.
- ❖ Reduce inflammation.
- ❖ Provide antimicrobial defense.
- ❖ Promote wound healing and decrease infection rate.
- ❖ Promote anti-aging benefits by increasing collagen production and reducing oxidative stress.

Foods Containing Probiotics

- ❖ *Fermented Dairy Products:* yogurt, kefir, traditional buttermilk.
- ❖ *Fermented Vegetables:* sauerkraut, kimchi, naturally fermented pickles (not those pickled with vinegar)
- ❖ *Fermented Soy Products:* miso, tempeh
- ❖ *Fermented Grains:* sourdough bread, fermented oats, such as overnight oats

Other Fermented Foods and Beverages:

- ❖ *Kombucha:* A fermented tea beverage that contains a variety of bacteria and yeast.
- ❖ *Kvass:* A traditional Eastern European fermented beverage made from rye bread.
- ❖ *Fermented Cheese:* Some types of aged cheese, such as Gouda, cheddar, and Swiss, can contain probiotics.
- ❖ *Probiotic Juices:* Some commercially available fruit and vegetable juices are fortified with probiotics.

Common Commercial Probiotics

Here is a list of common probiotics that are used for their beneficial effects on digestion, the immune system, skin, and other body systems.

Lactobacillus acidophilus

Lactobacillus acidophilus is one of the most common commercial probiotics.

It is naturally found in the human gastrointestinal tract, mouth, and vagina, and it is also present in various fermented foods like yogurt, kefir, and certain cheeses.

It produces lactic acid in the gastrointestinal tract, which creates an acidic environment that inhibits the growth of harmful bacteria.

It supports digestion by breaking down lactose, thus helping those with lactose intolerance, and enhances nutrient absorption.

Additionally, L. acidophilus helps alleviate symptoms of gastrointestinal disorders such as irritable bowel syndrome (IBS) and inflammatory bowel disease (IBD).

Its presence in the vaginal microbiome also helps maintain a healthy balance, preventing yeast infections and bacterial vaginosis.

Bifidobacterium

Bifidobacterium is naturally found in the human gastrointestinal tract, particularly in the colon, as well as in the mouth and vagina. It is also present in fermented foods like yogurt, kefir, and certain cheeses. It is also helpful for those suffering from irritable bowel syndrome (IBS) and inflammatory bowel disease (IBD).

Saccharomyces boulardii

Saccharomyces boulardii is actually a beneficial yeast and not a bacterium. It is particularly effective in preventing and treating various forms of diarrhea, including antibiotic-associated diarrhea, traveler's diarrhea, and diarrhea caused by Clostridium difficile infection. It also helps with IBS and IBD.

Streptococcus thermophilus

Streptococcus thermophilus is also found in fermented dairy products like yogurt and cheese. It aids in the breakdown of lactose, making it particularly beneficial for individuals with lactose intolerance. It also boosts the immune system, reduces inflammation, and prevents the translocation of harmful substances from the gut into the bloodstream.

How to Choose Probiotics

A probiotic strain is a specific type of bacteria or yeast within a species that has unique properties and health benefits. Probiotics are generally classified by their genus, species, and strain, for example, Lactobacillus (genus), acidophilus (species), and NCFM (strain). Each strain can have different effects on the body, even within the same species, due to variations in its genetic makeup and functions.

Choosing the right probiotic strain depends on various factors, including your specific health needs, the evidence supporting the strain's efficacy, and how well it can survive and thrive in your body. This means it can survive the acidic environment of the stomach and reach the intestines alive. Some probiotics require refrigeration to maintain their potency, while others are shelf-stable. Follow the storage instructions provided by the manufacturer to ensure the probiotics remain effective.

The potency of probiotics is measured in CFUs, which indicate the number of live microorganisms in each dose. The appropriate CFU count can vary depending on the strain and the health condition being targeted. Common CFU ranges for effective probiotic supplements are between 1 billion and 10 billion CFUs per day, but higher doses may be necessary for certain conditions.

Core Probiotic Strains that are commonly recommended for skin health include *Lactobacillus Rhamnosus GG, Lactobacillus Acidophilus, Lactobacillus Plantarum, Bifidobacterium Lactis (BB-12), Bifidobacterium Longum, Bifidobacterium Breve.*

At our clinic, we usually recommend multi-strain probiotic supplements, which contain a combination of different probiotic strains. These supplements can provide a broader range of benefits for multiple health concerns simultaneously. We personalize these recommendations based on patients' skin diseases and non-skin medical conditions.

Who Should Not Take Supplemental Probiotics?

While probiotics are generally considered safe for most people, certain groups should be cautious with probiotic supplementation:

People with Weakened Immune Systems

Individuals with compromised immune systems, such as those undergoing chemotherapy, people with HIV/AIDS, or patients on immunosuppressive drugs, are at higher risk for infections. There have been rare cases where probiotics have led to infections like bacteremia or fungemia in immunocompromised patients.

Individuals with Severe Illnesses

Those with severe or critical illnesses, especially those in intensive care units (ICU), should avoid probiotics due to the increased risk of infections. In these patients, probiotics can potentially translocate across the gut barrier and cause sepsis or other serious infections.

Individuals with Known Allergies to Probiotic Components

As always, please consult your clinician about the probiotic regimen, strains, and dosages.

Prebiotics

Simply put, prebiotics are non-digestible fibers that serve as the food for probiotics. Like probiotics, prebiotics could be found in common foods or could be taken supplementally.

Foods Containing Prebiotics:

- ❖ *Fibrous Vegetables:* Onions, garlic, leeks, asparagus, artichokes, and chicory root.
- ❖ *Fruits:* Bananas, apples, and berries.
- ❖ *Whole Grains:* Oats, barley, and whole wheat.
- ❖ *Legumes:* Lentils, chickpeas, and beans.
- ❖ *Nuts and Seeds:* Flaxseeds and chia seeds.

Common Commercial Prebiotics

The prebiotics below are available as powders or capsules.

- ❖ *Inulin* is found in chicory root, Jerusalem artichokes, and other plants. It promotes the growth of beneficial bacteria such as Bifidobacteria and Lactobacilli, improves digestion, and helps regulate bowel movements.
- ❖ *Fructooligosaccharides (FOS)* are found naturally in fruits and vegetables like bananas, onions, and garlic. They improve mineral absorption (e.g., calcium).
- ❖ *Galactooligosaccharides (GOS)* are derived from lactose, commonly found in dairy products. They reduce the risk of infections.
- ❖ **Resistant Starch** is in foods such as green bananas, potatoes, and grains that have been cooked and cooled. It improves insulin sensitivity and supports digestive health.
- ❖ *Psyllium Husk* is derived from the seeds of the Plantago ovata plant. It promotes regular bowel movements, supports overall digestive health, and helps maintain healthy blood sugar levels.

- *Acacia Fiber* is derived from the sap of the Acacia tree. It supports the growth of beneficial bacteria, helps with digestive health, and can aid in weight management.
- *Isomaltooligosaccharides (IMO)* are found in fermented foods and some plants. They promote bowel regularity.
- *Lactulose* is synthetic sugar derived from lactose. It is used primarily to treat constipation and hepatic encephalopathy by promoting the growth of beneficial gut bacteria.

Who Should Avoid Supplemental Prebiotics?

People with Sensitivity to FODMAPs

You may have recognized the "saccharides" component in the names of many prebiotics, as we saw earlier in Chapter 15, *FODMAP Sensitivity and Skin Conditions*. Indeed, many prebiotics are high FODMAP foods, so despite their beneficial qualities, they will have to be removed from your diet if you have sensitivities to FODMAPs.

Individuals with Irritable Bowel Syndrome (IBS)

Prebiotics, particularly those high in FODMAPs, can exacerbate symptoms of IBS, such as gas production, bloating, abdominal pain, and diarrhea.

People with Small Intestinal Bacterial Overgrowth (SIBO)

SIBO involves an abnormal increase in the population of bacteria in the small intestine, where bacteria are usually present in lower numbers. Prebiotics can further feed these bacteria, worsening symptoms like bloating, abdominal pain, and diarrhea.

People with Fructose Malabsorption

Many prebiotics are fructo-oligosaccharides (FOS), which are chains of fructose molecules.

Individuals with fructose malabsorption may experience gastrointestinal distress.

Individuals with Certain Food Allergies or Intolerances to the components of prebiotics supplements.

Glutamine

Glutamine is the most abundant amino acid in the human body, and 60% of our muscles are made from it. It is not surprising that it serves as a building block for proteins, playing a crucial role in muscle maintenance and growth. Glutamine is a primary fuel source for the gut cells and plays an important role in preserving gut permeability.

Although glutamine is classified as a non-essential amino acid because the body can produce it, it becomes conditionally essential during periods of intense physical stress or trauma as the body's demand for glutamine increases significantly. Glutamine is vital for muscle recovery.

Effects of Glutamine on Skin

- ❖ Promotes Wound Healing through cell proliferation and the synthesis of proteins and collagen, which are crucial for wound repair and tissue regeneration.
- ❖ Maintains Skin Barrier Function by protecting it from infections.

- Keeps skin hydrated by preventing water loss.
- Helps reduce skin inflammation, which is especially important in eczema and psoriasis.
- Contributes to the synthesis of glutathione, a potent antioxidant that protects skin cells from oxidative damage.
- Takes part in the synthesis of hyaluronic acid and other compounds that maintain skin hydration and elasticity.

Food Sources of Glutamine:

- *Animal Proteins:* Beef, pork, chicken, salmon, cod, mackerel, shellfish, both egg whites and yolks
- *Dairy Products:* milk, Greek yogurt, cottage cheese, ricotta
- *Plant-Based Sources:* beans, lentils, peas, almonds, walnuts, sunflower seeds, peanuts, spinach, cabbage, beets, and parsley.
- *Grains:* wheat bread and rice, corn

Who Should Take Glutamine Supplements?

Glutamine supplements can be beneficial for various groups of people, particularly those with increased physiological demands or specific health conditions, for example:

Athletes and Bodybuilders

Glutamine helps in muscle repair and reduces muscle soreness after intense exercise. Also, strenuous physical activity can suppress the immune system; glutamine supports immune function, reducing the risk of illness post-exercise.

Individuals with Gastrointestinal Disorders, such as IBS and leaky gut.

Glutamine supports the gut lining that is damaged in these GI disorders.

Post-Surgery and Trauma Patients

Glutamine is crucial for cell proliferation and the synthesis of proteins and collagen, aiding in faster wound recovery and healing. It also supports the immune system during recovery from surgery or traumatic injuries.

People with Chronic Stress

Chronic stress depletes glutamine levels, impacting immune function and gut health. Supplementation can help restore these levels and mitigate the effects of stress.

Individuals with Metabolic Stress

Conditions like sepsis or severe infections can increase the body's demand for glutamine. Supplementation can support the body's recovery by providing the necessary amino acids for metabolic functions.

Who Should Avoid Glutamine Supplements?

- Individuals with Liver Disease
- People with Kidney Disease
- Individuals with Seizure Disorder
- People with Bipolar Disorder
- Pregnant and Breastfeeding Women
- Individuals with Sensitivity or Allergic Reactions

As always, please consult with a healthcare professional before starting any new supplements, especially if you have existing health conditions or are taking other medications.

Collagen

Collagen is the most abundant protein in the human body, making up about a third of its protein composition. It's a major component of your connective tissues, including skin, hair, nails, bones, muscles, and ligaments. The primary amino acids in collagen are proline, glycine, and hydroxyproline. The role of collagen in skin health is intertwined with its impact on joints and bones, so let's look at all of them.

There are many types of collagens, but the most pertinent ones are:

- Type I. The most abundant type of collagen in the body contributes to skin, bones, tendons, and vascular structures.
- Type II is found in the cartilage of joints.
- Type III is in the skin, lungs, and intestinal walls.
- Type IV comprises the layers of skin.
- Type V is found in the skin, cornea, and placenta.

Effect of Collagen on Skin, Joints and Bone:

- *Supports skin youthfulness:* Collagen reduces wrinkles by enhancing skin elasticity and hydration.
- *Supports Joint Health:* Collagen helps maintain the integrity of your cartilage, the tissue that protects your joints. It can reduce joint pain and improve joint mobility.

- ❖ **_Strengthens Hair and Nails:_** Collagen can improve the strength and growth of your hair and nails by reducing brittleness and breakage while adding shine to hair.
- ❖ **_Supports Bone Health:_** Collagen enhances bone density, reducing the risk of osteoporosis and fractures as you age.

As we age, the body's ability to produce collagen decreases. This reduction typically starts in the mid-20s and accelerates in the following decades. Reduced collagen levels can lead to signs of aging such as wrinkles, sagging skin, joint pain, loss of muscle tissues, etc.

Food Sources of Collagen:

Bone Broth: It provides a direct source of collagen along with amino acids like glycine and proline, which are essential for collagen synthesis.

Meat and poultry, fish and shellfish, eggs, dairy products.

Types of Collagen Supplements

Collagen supplements are often made as a tasteless powder that can be added to smoothies, coffee, or any beverage.

The popular form of collagen is *collagen peptides*, which is a form of collagen that has been broken into smaller pieces (peptides) to help with ingestion. These collagen peptides are usually derived from cows or pigs.

Marine Collagen, sourced from fish, is especially beneficial for improving skin hydration, enhancing elasticity, and reducing wrinkles.

It is particularly rich in Type I collagen. Yet, it may have a fishy taste, and you can't take it if you are allergic to fish or shellfish.

In general, collagen supplements are generally safe for most people. Potential side effects may include mild digestive issues, such as bloating or gas.

If you're pregnant, breastfeeding, or have any underlying health conditions, talk to your clinician before starting collagen supplements.

Omega-3 Fatty Acids

Omega-3 fatty acids are essential fats that your body needs but cannot produce on its own. They are crucial for many bodily functions, including brain and heart health. To put it simply, they decrease inflammation throughout the body.

There are three main types of omega-3 fatty acids: **EPA (Eicosapentaenoic Acid)**, **DHA (Docosahexaenoic Acid)** and **ALA (Alpha-Linolenic Acid)**

The benefits of omega-3 fatty acids include lowering blood pressure and triglycerides, supporting brain function (DHA), and reducing inflammation in chronic diseases like arthritis.

The Effects of Omega-3 Fatty Acids on Skin:

- ❖ *Anti-Inflammatory Properties:* They reduce inflammation, which is an essential component of inflammatory conditions such as acne, psoriasis, and eczema.
- ❖ *Skin Barrier Function:* Omega-3 fatty acids help maintain the skin lipid barrier, which is crucial for retaining

moisture and protecting against external irritants. This helps keep the skin hydrated and reduces dryness and irritation.

- ❖ **Protection Against UV Damage:** Omega-3 fatty acids can help protect the skin from the harmful effects of UV radiation by reducing inflammation and supporting skin repair mechanisms. So, they help mitigate the effects of sun exposure, reducing the risk of sunburn and long-term damage that can lead to premature aging and skin cancer.
- ❖ **Enhanced Skin Healing:** They play a role in cell membrane health and repair, promoting quicker and more effective healing of skin injuries. This results in quicker recovery from wounds, cuts, and other injuries more efficiently, reducing the risk of infection and scarring.

Recommended Dosages of Omega-3 Fatty Acids

American Heart Association Recommended Dosages of Omega-3 Fatty Acids in Healthy Adults Without Heart Disease

EPA and DHA: 500 mg per day combined EPA and DHA.

ALA: 1.6 grams per day for men and 1.1 grams per day for women.

Food Sources of Omega-3 Fatty Acids:

- ❖ **Fish and Seafood (EPA and DHA):** salmon, mackerel, sardines, anchovies, herring, tuna.
- ❖ **Plant-Based Sources (ALA):** flaxseeds, chia seeds, hemp seeds, walnuts.

Oils

- ❖ **Fish Oil**: High in EPA and DHA. It is derived from the tissues of oily fish, such as salmon, mackerel, and sardines.
- ❖ **Cod Liver Oil**: Contains EPA, DHA, and vitamins A and D. Extracted from the liver of codfish.
- ❖ **Krill Oil**: Contains EPA and DHA, along with a powerful antioxidant called astaxanthin. Made from tiny crustaceans called krill.
- ❖ **Algal Oil**: Rich in DHA, some formulations also contain EPA. Suitable for vegetarians and vegans.
- ❖ **Flaxseed Oil**: High in ALA, which the body can convert to EPA and DHA at a lower conversion rate. Extracted from flaxseeds. Suitable for vegetarians and vegans.

Using supplements containing both EPA and DHA is preferable for whole health and skin health in particular.

Omega-3 fatty acids supplements come in the form of softgels, liquids, and gummies.

The Risks of Omega-3 Fatty Acids Supplements:

- ❖ **Bleeding Risk**: High doses of omega-3s can increase bleeding risk due to their blood-thinning effects. People on blood-thinning medications should consult their healthcare provider before taking omega-3 supplements. It is usually recommended to stop omega-3s prior to major procedures.
- ❖ **Gastrointestinal Issues**: Omega-3s may cause indigestion, nausea, diarrhea, or fishy aftertaste.

- ❖ ***Potential Contaminants:*** Fish oil supplements can contain contaminants like mercury, polychlorinated biphenyls (PCBs), and dioxins. Choose high-quality, purified products that are third-party tested for purity.
- ❖ ***Allergic Reactions:*** People with fish or shellfish allergies may react to fish oil or krill oil supplements. Please note that some fish oil supplements may contain soy.

CHAPTER 23

Clear Skin Lifestyle

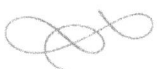

Achieving clear, healthy skin isn't just about the foods you eat—though diet plays a crucial role. Your lifestyle, including how you manage stress, the quality of your sleep, the amount of exercise you get, and the connections you maintain with others, can significantly influence the health of your skin. I often notice that patients focus on removing food sensitivities and changing their diet but are reluctant to make other changes as they don't perceive them to be directly related to their skin. I hope this book, with its sections on the effects of cortisol—a stress hormone—on various skin conditions, has dispelled that myth. Cortisol doesn't act alone; it also influences other hormones and impacts our gut health. So, a clear skin diet is also a mindful diet (in addition to being a gut-friendly diet).

Components of Clear Skin Diet are mindful eating, stress-reducing activities, good sleep, exercise and healthy and positive and meaningful connections.

Mindful Eating

Mindful eating is the practice of paying full attention to the experience of eating and drinking, both inside and outside the body. How does it help?

Enhances Digestion Through Relaxation

Mindful eating encourages a relaxed state during meals. When you're relaxed, your parasympathetic nervous system, often referred to as the "rest and digest" system, is activated. This state promotes optimal digestion by increasing blood flow to the digestive organs, enhancing the production of digestive enzymes, and facilitating the smooth movement of food through the digestive tract.

Improves Chewing and Saliva Production

Mindful eating involves thoroughly chewing food, which is the first step in the digestive process. Proper chewing breaks down food into smaller particles, making it easier for stomach acids and enzymes to digest it further. Additionally, the act of chewing stimulates saliva production. Saliva contains digestive enzymes like amylase, which begins the breakdown of carbohydrates in the mouth, easing the digestive workload on the stomach and intestines.

Improves Awareness of Hunger and Fullness Cues

Mindful eating helps you tune into your body's natural hunger and fullness signals, preventing overeating or eating when you're not truly hungry. Overeating can overload the digestive system, leading to discomfort, indigestion, and bloating. By listening to your body's cues, you can avoid these issues and give your digestive system the right amount of food to process.

Reduces Digestive Discomfort

Eating mindfully means slowing down and savoring each bite. This slower pace can prevent common digestive issues like acid reflux, indigestion, and bloating, often exacerbated by eating too quickly. When you eat slowly, you give your body time to properly signal when it's full, reducing the risk of overeating and the associated digestive discomfort.

Increases Nutrient Absorption

Mindful eating encourages you to focus on the sensory experience of eating—the taste, texture, and aroma of your food. This heightened awareness can lead to better food choices, often favoring nutrient-dense, whole foods over processed options. Additionally, because you're chewing more thoroughly and allowing your body to digest food at its own pace, your body can more effectively absorb and utilize the nutrients in your food.

Provides Emotional and Psychological Benefits

Stress and negative emotions can interfere with digestion, often leading to issues like irritable bowel syndrome (IBS) and other digestive disorders. Mindful eating helps reduce stress and promotes a positive relationship with food, which can alleviate these issues. Being present and enjoying your meal can reduce the emotional triggers that might otherwise disrupt your digestion.

Mindful Eating Practices for Improved Digestion

Here are some simple ways to incorporate mindful eating into your routine to support digestion:

- ❖ *Sit Down and Eat Without Distractions:* Focus on your meal without the distractions of TV, smartphones, or work. This allows you to fully engage with the experience of eating.
- ❖ *Take Small Bites and Chew Thoroughly: Chew* each bite slowly and completely before swallowing. This practice helps your body begin the digestive process in the mouth and reduces the workload on your stomach and intestines.
- ❖ *Pause Between Bites:* Put your utensils down between bites and take a moment to breathe and appreciate the food. This can help you eat more slowly and recognize when you're comfortably full.
- ❖ *Listen to Your Body:* Pay attention to your body's signals of hunger and fullness. Eat when you're hungry and stop when you're satisfied, not overly full.
- ❖ *Express Gratitude for Your Food:* Taking a moment to appreciate your meal can enhance your connection to the food and the eating experience, promoting a more positive and relaxed approach to eating.

Examples of Stress-Reducing Activities

Yoga

Yoga consists of physical postures, breathing exercises, and meditation, making it a powerful tool for reducing stress. It helps release tension from the body, while the mindfulness aspect promotes relaxation and stress relief.

Journaling

Writing down your thoughts and feelings can be a therapeutic way to manage stress. Journaling allows you to process emotions and gain perspective on stressful situations, which can reduce their impact on your skin.

Nature Walks

Spending time in nature can be incredibly grounding and soothing. Walking in a park, forest, or by the ocean can help lower stress levels and provide your skin with a natural glow due to improved circulation and oxygenation.

Creative Outlets

Engaging in creative activities such as painting, drawing, or playing music can be a great way to unwind and reduce stress. These activities can help shift your focus away from stressors and allow your body to relax.

The Importance of Good Sleep

Sleep is often referred to as "beauty sleep" for a reason. During sleep, your body goes into repair mode, healing, and regenerating cells, including those in your skin. Lack of sleep can lead to dull skin, dark circles, and increased signs of aging. Prioritizing good sleep hygiene is essential for maintaining clear and vibrant skin.

Tips for Improving Sleep Quality:

- *Maintain a Regular Sleep Schedule:* Going to bed and waking up at the same time every day helps regulate your body's internal clock, making it easier to fall asleep and wake up refreshed. Consistency in your sleep schedule also ensures that your body gets the rest it needs for skin repair.
- *Create a Relaxing Bedtime Routine:* Establishing a calming routine before bed can signal to your body that it's time to wind down. Activities such as reading, taking a warm bath, or practicing gentle stretches can help prepare your mind and body for sleep.
- *Optimize Your Sleep Environment:* Your bedroom should be a sleep sanctuary. Keep the room cool, dark, and quiet. Investing in a comfortable mattress and pillows can also make a significant difference in the quality of your sleep.
- *Limit Screen Time Before Bed:* The blue light emitted from phones, tablets, and computers can interfere with your body's production of melatonin, the hormone that regulates sleep. Try to avoid screens at least an hour before bedtime to ensure a better night's sleep.
- *Practice Relaxation Techniques:* If you have trouble falling asleep, consider practicing relaxation techniques such as deep breathing, progressive muscle relaxation, or visualization. These techniques can help calm your mind and prepare your body for restful sleep.

Exercise

Regular physical activity is not only beneficial for your overall health but also plays a significant role in maintaining clear skin. Exercise increases blood flow, which helps nourish skin cells and keeps them vital. It also helps reduce stress, regulate hormones, and improve sleep—all of which contribute to healthier skin.

Types of Exercises for Healthy Skin:

- *Cardiovascular Exercise:* Activities like running, swimming, cycling, and dancing increase your heart rate and improve circulation. Better circulation means more oxygen and nutrients are delivered to your skin, promoting a healthy glow and aiding in removing toxins.
- *Strength Training:* Lifting weights or performing bodyweight exercises helps build muscle and burn fat. Strength training can also balance hormones, which is crucial for preventing acne and other skin issues related to hormonal imbalances.
- *Yoga and Pilates:* These exercises combine strength, flexibility, and mindfulness, making them excellent for stress reduction and improving skin health. The deep breathing and stretching involved in these practices enhance blood flow and promote relaxation.
- *High-Intensity Interval Training (HIIT):* HIIT workouts, which alternate between short bursts of intense exercise and rest periods, are efficient at improving cardiovascu-

lar health, burning calories, and regulating hormones, all of which can contribute to clearer skin.

- ❖ *Outdoor Activities:* Exercising outdoors, such as hiking, running, or playing sports, exposes your skin to fresh air and sunlight. Just be sure to protect your skin with sunscreen to avoid sun damage.

Positive and Meaningful Connections

Human beings are social creatures, and our connections with others can profoundly impact our mental and physical health, including the health of our skin. Positive relationships and social interactions can reduce stress, boost mood, and improve overall well-being, leading to healthier skin.

Ways to Cultivate Positive Connections:

- ❖ *Build Strong Relationships:* Cultivating meaningful relationships with family, friends, and partners can provide emotional support and reduce stress. Strong social connections are linked to better health outcomes, including healthier skin.
- ❖ *Engage in Social Activities:* Participating in group activities, clubs, or community events can help you build new connections and strengthen existing ones. Socializing in a positive environment can boost your mood and reduce the impact of stress on your skin.
- ❖ *Practice Active Listening:* Being present and truly listening to others can deepen your relationships and reduce misunderstandings. Positive communication can

enhance your emotional well-being and contribute to a healthy, glowing complexion.

- ❖ ***Seek Support When Needed:*** If you're going through a challenging time, don't hesitate to reach out to friends, family, or a professional for support. Talking through your feelings can alleviate stress and prevent its negative effects on your skin.
- ❖ ***Nurture Self-Compassion***: While connecting with others is important, having a healthy relationship with yourself is equally crucial. Practicing self-compassion and self-care can reduce stress and help you maintain clear, healthy skin.

CONCLUSION

Achieving clear, radiant skin is about much more than just the products you use on the surface; it's a holistic journey that begins with what you nourish your body with and how you live your life. In this book, we've explored the powerful connection between food sensitivities and skin health, providing you with the knowledge and tools to take control of your skin from the inside out.

In Part I, we started by demystifying food sensitivities and their distinct differences from food allergies. This foundational knowledge sets the stage for making informed decisions leading to healthier, clearer skin.

Part II took us deeper into the science behind how food sensitivities can trigger skin conditions. We explored the immune system's role in inflammation, the impact of histamine release, and the critical connection between gut health and skin health. By understanding these mechanisms, you gain insight into how your body responds to certain foods and how these responses can manifest in your skin. This holistic perspective highlights the importance of treating the body as an interconnected system, where every part plays a role in your overall well-being.

Conclusion

In Part III, we examined specific food sensitivities and their direct impact on the skin. We discussed how these common triggers can lead to various skin conditions and provided practical strategies for managing them. Armed with this knowledge, you can make dietary choices that support your skin's health, helping you avoid potential triggers and embrace foods that promote clear, glowing skin.

Part IV focused on practical tools for identifying food sensitivities, including food diaries, elimination diets, and testing methods. These tools are essential for anyone looking to pinpoint the foods that may be causing their skin issues. By methodically testing and eliminating potential triggers, you can create a personalized diet that supports your skin's needs and promotes long-term health.

In the final section, Part V, we offered a comprehensive guide to the Clear Skin Diet and the lifestyle changes that can support your journey to better skin. We emphasized the importance of a balanced diet rich in whole foods, fiber, vitamins, minerals, and key supplements like probiotics, prebiotics, and omega-3 fatty acids. We also discussed lifestyle factors like mindful eating, stress management, quality sleep, regular exercise, and maintaining positive social connections—all of which are vital to achieving and maintaining healthy skin.

The Clear Skin Diet is not a one-size-fits-all solution; it's a personalized journey that requires careful attention to your body's unique needs. By applying the knowledge and strategies from this book, you can take meaningful steps toward improving your skin health, reducing the impact of food sensitivities, and achieving the clear, radiant skin you desire.

REFERENCES

Introduction

Part I. Food Sensitivities and Skin Health: Definitions and Key Concepts

Bowe WP, Joshi SS. Diet and dermatology: the role of dietary intervention in skin disease. J Clin Aesthet Dermatol. 2020;13(12):46-52.

Zhang Y, Cai W, Zhou L, Liu S, Zhao Y, Zhao W. Food sensitivities: Mechanisms, manifestations, and management strategies. Nutr Rev. 2021;79(10):1131-1146.

Parker M, Romano C, Gambineri E. The gut-skin axis: implications for skin health and disease. J Eur Acad Dermatol Venereol. 2022;36(8):1247-1256.

Mills EN, Sancho AI, Rigby NM, Jenkins JA, Mackie AR. Impact of food structure on allergenicity. Trends Food Sci Technol. 2020; 102:104-113.

Rinaldi M, Perricone R, Blank M, Perricone C, Shoenfeld Y. Anti-food antibodies in the diagnosis of food allergy: Is it time to start using them? J Clin Immunol. 2021;41(4):757-765.

Francisco V, Ruiz-Fernández C, Pino J, et al. Dietary inflammatory index and skin diseases: a systematic review and meta-analysis. Nutrients. 2021;13(3):857.

Castaldo G, Izzo L, Troiano A, et al. Functional foods and nutraceuticals in the management of skin health: a review. Molecules. 2020;25(21):5107.

References

Kim SY, Kim JH, Lee YJ, Park JW, Kim SH. Oral food challenge for the diagnosis of food allergy. J Korean Med Sci. 2021;36(7)

Tsakok T, Woolf R, Smith CH, Weidinger S. Atopic dermatitis: the skin barrier, microbiome, and new therapies. J Allergy Clin Immunol. 2019;143(6):2045-2055.

DeMartin S, Guillet G, Thomas L, et al. The role of diet in the prevention and treatment of acne: a review of the literature. J Eur Acad Dermatol Venereol. 2020;34(2):225-230.

Zaenglein AL, Pathy AL, Schlosser BJ, et al. Guidelines of care for the management of acne vulgaris. J Am Acad Dermatol. 2016;74(5):945-973.e33.

Nutten S. Atopic dermatitis: global epidemiology and risk factors. Ann Nutr Metab. 2015;66(Suppl 1):8-16.

Picardo M, Eichenfield LF, Tan J. Acne and rosacea. Dermatol Ther (Heidelb). 2017;7(Suppl 1):43-52.

Turner GA, Hoptroff M, Harding CR. Stratum corneum dysfunction in dandruff. Int J Cosmet Sci. 2012;34(4):298-306.

Johansen JD, Aalto-Korte K, Agner T, et al. European Society of Contact Dermatitis guideline for diagnostic patch testing – recommendations on best practice. Contact Dermatitis. 2015;73(4):195-221.

Griffiths CE, van de Kerkhof P, Czarnecka-Operacz M. Psoriasis and atopic dermatitis. Dermatol Ther (Heidelb). 2017;7(Suppl 1):31-41.

Thibaut de Schotten T, Roujeau JC. Rosacea: an update on diagnosis and treatment. J Eur Acad Dermatol Venereol. 2020;34(3):508-515.

Vestergaard C, Deleuran M. The pathophysiology of urticaria. Immunol Allergy Clin North Am. 2014;34(1):15-24.

Sørensen SBT, Farkas DK, Vestergaard C, Schmidt SAJ, Lindahl LM, Mansfield KE, et al. Urticaria and the risk of cancer: a Danish population-based cohort study. Br J Dermatol. 2024 Jun 27

Balp MM, Lopes M, Benmedjahed K, et al. The impact of pruritus in patients with psoriasis: results from the UPLIFT survey. J Eur Acad Dermatol Venereol. 2018;32(12):2220-2227.

Part II. Mechanism of Action: How Food Sensitivities May Cause Skin Conditions

Chen L, Deng H, Cui H, et al. Inflammatory responses and inflammation-associated diseases in organs. Oncotarget. 2018;9(6):7204-7218.

Zhang JM, An J. Cytokines, inflammation, and pain. Int Anesthesiol Clin. 2007;45(2):27-37.

Dinarello CA. Overview of the IL-1 family in innate inflammation and acquired immunity. Immunol Rev. 2018;281(1):8-27.

Ricciotti E, FitzGerald GA. Prostaglandins and inflammation. Arterioscler Thromb Vasc Biol. 2011;31(5):986-1000.

Samuelsson B. Arachidonic acid metabolism: role in inflammation. Z Ernahrungswiss. 1988;27(1):1-12.

Serhan CN, Hamberg M, Samuelsson B. Lipoxins: novel series of biologically active compounds formed from arachidonic acid in human leukocytes. Proc Natl Acad Sci USA. 1984;81(17):5335-5339.

Levy BD, Serhan CN. Resolution of acute inflammation in the lung. Annu Rev Physiol. 2014; 76:467-492.

Gilroy DW, Bishop-Bailey D. Lipid mediators in immune regulation and resolution. Br J Pharmacol. 2019;176(8):1009-1023.

Montuschi P, Peters-Golden M. Leukotriene modifiers for asthma treatment. Clin Exp Allergy. 2020;50(8):965-974.

Kim SH, Urao N. Prostaglandins in skin wound healing. Int J Mol Sci. 2019;20(19):5023.

Afrin LB, Butterfield JH, Raithel M, Molderings GJ. Often seen, rarely recognized: mast cell activation disease—a guide to diagnosis and therapeutic options. Ann Med. 2016;48(3):190-201.

References

Comas-Basté O, Sánchez-Pérez S, Veciana-Nogués MT, et al. Histamine intolerance: the current state of the art. Biomolecules. 2020;10(8):1181.

Maintz L, Novak N. Histamine and histamine intolerance. Am J Clin Nutr. 2007;85(5):1185-1196.

Theoharides TC, Valent P, Akin C. Mast cells, mastocytosis, and related disorders. N Engl J Med. 2015;373(2):1885-1886.

Kovacova-Hanuskova E, Buday T, Gavliakova S, Plevkova J. Histamine, histamine intoxication and intolerance. Allergol Immunopathol (Madr). 2015;43(5):498-506.

Friedlaender GE. The histamine H4 receptor: a promising target for the treatment of allergic disorders. J Allergy Clin Immunol. 2014;134(4):722-729.

Manzotti G, Breda D, Di Gioacchino M, Burastero SE. Serum diamine oxidase activity in patients with histamine intolerance. Int J Immunopathol Pharmacol. 2016;29(1):105-111.

Frieri M, Patel R, Celestin J. Mast cell activation syndrome: a review. Curr Allergy Asthma Rep. 2013;13(1):27-32.

Kaur RJ, Khan DA, Mutasim DF. Mast cell activation syndrome: an update. Dermatitis. 2021;32(3):182-189.

Jarisch R. Histamine intolerance in dermatology. Am J Clin Dermatol. 2004;5(5):327-330.

Fasano A. Leaky gut and autoimmune diseases. Clin Rev Allergy Immunol. 2012;42(1):71-78.

Turnbaugh PJ, Ley RE, Hamady M, et al. The human microbiome project. Nature. 2007;449(7164):804-810.

El-Serag HB, Sweet S, Winchester CC, Dent J. Update on the epidemiology of gastro-oesophageal reflux disease: a systematic review. Gut. 2014;63(6):871-880.

Camilleri M, Lasch K, Zhou W. Irritable bowel syndrome: methods, mechanisms, and pathophysiology. The confluence of increased permeability, inflammation, and pain in irritable bowel syndrome. Am J Physiol Gastrointest Liver Physiol. 2012;303(7)

Arrieta MC, Bistritz L, Meddings JB. Alterations in intestinal permeability. Gut. 2006;55(10):1512-1520.

Rieder R, Wisniewski PJ, Alderman BL, Campbell SC. Microbes and mental health: A review. Brain Behav Immun. 2017;66:9-17.

Sturgeon C, Fasano A. Zonulin, a regulator of epithelial and endothelial barrier functions, and its involvement in chronic inflammatory diseases. Tissue Barriers. 2016;4(4)

.Mayer EA, Tillisch K, Gupta A. Gut/brain axis and the microbiota. J Clin Invest. 2015;125(3):926-938.

Bischoff SC. 'Gut health': a new objective in medicine? BMC Med. 2011;9:24.

Wang Y, Kasper LH. The role of microbiome in central nervous system disorders. Brain Behav Immun. 2014;38:1-12.

Veres-Székely A, Szász C, Pap D, Szebeni B, Bokrossy P, Vannay Á. Zonulin as a potential therapeutic target in microbiota-gut-brain axis disorders: encouraging results and emerging questions. Int J Mol Sci. 2023;24(8):7548.

Smith TM, Gillman MW, Mailick MR, et al. Insulin-like growth factor-1 and acne vulgaris: a cohort-based study. J Invest Dermatol. 2007;127(9):2148-2153.

Melnik BC. Milk consumption: aggravating factor of acne and promoter of chronic diseases of Western societies. J Dtsch Dermatol Ges. 2009;7(4):364-370.

Thiboutot D. Acne: hormonal concepts and therapy. Clin Dermatol. 2004;22(5):419-428.

Du X, Xu Y. Insulin-like growth factor-1, androgen, and acne: new insights from studies of pluripotent stem cells. J Invest Dermatol. 2021;141(8):2010-2014.

Brand JS, Chan MF, Dowsett M, et al. Testosterone, SHBG and the development of acne in adolescent girls and boys. Clin Endocrinol (Oxf). 2021;94(1):155-163.

Rosenfield RL. The relationship of excessive adrenal and ovarian androgen secretion to the pathogenesis of polycystic ovarian syndrome. J Endocrinol Invest. 2019;42(6):701-708.

Pekmezci E. Phytoestrogens and health. J Med Food. 2019;22(10):1029-1036.

Peeters PH, Keinan-Boker L, Van der Schouw YT, Grobbee DE. Phytoestrogens and breast cancer risk: review of the epidemiological evidence. Breast Cancer Res Treat. 2003;77(2):171-183.

Leung AKC, Barankin B, Hon KL. Physiological skin changes in pregnancy. Am Fam Physician. 2016;94(3):211-215.

Hennessey JV. Diagnosis and management of thyrotoxicosis. Am Fam Physician. 2015;91(6):362-368.

Part III. Common Food Sensitivities and Their Skin Effects

Fasano A, Catassi C. Current approaches to diagnosis and treatment of celiac disease: an evolving spectrum. Gastroenterology. 2001;120(3):636-651.

Sapone A, Bai JC, Ciacci C, et al. Spectrum of gluten-related disorders: consensus on new nomenclature and classification. BMC Med. 2012; 10:13.

Green PH, Cellier C. Celiac disease. N Engl J Med. 2007;357(17):1731-1743.

Hadjivassiliou M, Sanders DS, Grünewald RA, Woodroofe N, Boscolo S, Aeschlimann D. Gluten sensitivity: from gut to brain. Lancet Neurol. 2010;9(3):318-330.

De Giorgio R, Volta U, Gibson PR, et al. Sensitivity to wheat, gluten and FODMAPs in IBS: facts or fiction? Gut. 2016;65(1):169-178.

Melnik BC. Milk consumption and acne: the role of IGF-1. J Am Acad Dermatol. 2011;65(1):59-66.

Vojdani A, O'Bryan T, Kellermann GH. The immunology of gluten sensitivity beyond the intestinal tract. Eur J Inflamm. 2008;6(2):177-189.

Catassi C, Bai JC, Bonaz B, et al. Non-celiac gluten sensitivity: the new frontier of gluten related disorders. Nutrients. 2013;5(10):3839-3853.

Cianferoni A, Spergel JM. Food allergy: review, classification and diagnosis. Allergol Int. 2009;58(4):457-466.

Ludvigsson JF, Bai JC, Biagi F, et al. Diagnosis and management of adult coeliac disease: guidelines from the British Society of Gastroenterology. Gut. 2014;63(8):1210-1228.

Messina M, Rogero MM, Fisberg M, Waitzberg D. Health implications of dietary soy protein and soy-derived isoflavones in postmenopausal women. J Nutr. 2017;147(11): 2322S-2336S.

Leung AM, Lamar A, He X, et al. Effect of soy protein isolate and soy phytoestrogens on thyroid function in healthy adults and adults with subclinical hypothyroidism: A randomized controlled trial. J Clin Endocrinol Metab. 2018;103(10):3821-3826.

Divi RL, Doerge DR. Inhibition of thyroid peroxidase by dietary flavonoids. Chem Res Toxicol. 1996;9(1):16-23.

Chen A, Chung E, Joung KE, et al. Soy food intake and breast cancer survival. JAMA. 2009;302(22):2437-2443.

Melnik BC, Schmitz G. Role of insulin, insulin-like growth factor-1, hyperglycaemic food and milk consumption in the pathogenesis of acne vulgaris. Exp Dermatol. 2009;18(10):833-841.

Melnik BC, John SM, Schmitz G. Over-stimulation of insulin/IGF-1 signaling by western diet may promote diseases of civilization: lessons learnt from Laron syndrome. Nutr Metab. 2011; 8:41.

Smith RN, Mann NJ, Braue A, Mäkeläinen H, Varigos GA. The effect of a high-protein, low glycemic-load diet versus a conventional, high glycemic-load diet on biochemical parameters associated with acne vulgaris: a randomized controlled trial. J Am Acad Dermatol. 2007;57(2):247-256.

Boelsma E, van de Vijver LP, Goldbohm RA, et al. Human skin condition and its associations with nutrient concentrations in serum and diet. Am J Clin Nutr. 2003;77(2):348-355.

Cohen DA, Story M. Sugar-sweetened beverages, artificial sweeteners, and obesity. Am J Public Health. 2014;104(4):616-618.

Fleming SE. Sugar, diet and skin conditions. In: Nutrition and Skin. Springer; 2011. p. 217-235.

World Health Organization. WHO advises not to use non-sugar sweeteners for weight control in newly released guideline. Geneva: World Health Organization; 2023.

Eggesbø M, Botten G, Halvorsen R, Magnus P. The prevalence of allergy to egg: a population-based study in young children. Allergy. 2001;56(5):403-411.

Savage JH, Matsui EC, Skripak JM, Wood RA. The natural history of egg allergy. J Allergy Clin Immunol. 2007;120(6):1413-1417.

Kelso JM, Greenhawt MJ, Li JT. Adverse reactions to vaccines practice parameter 2012 update. J Allergy Clin Immunol. 2012;130(1):25-43.

Warren CM, Jiang J, Gupta RS. Epidemiology and burden of food allergy. Curr Allergy Asthma Rep. 2020;20(2):6.

Teuber SS, Peterson WR. Systemic allergic reactions to hazelnut, walnut, and cashew in a birch-pollen-hypersensitive patient. J Allergy Clin Immunol. 1999;103(6):1285-1288.

Venter C, Maslin K, Patil V, et al. Prevalence and cumulative incidence of food hypersensitivity in the first 10 years of life. Pediatr Allergy Immunol. 2016;27(5):452-458.

Sicherer SH, Sampson HA. Peanut allergy: emerging concepts and approaches for an apparent epidemic. J Allergy Clin Immunol. 2007;120(3):491-503.

Hu FB, Stampfer MJ, Manson JE, et al. Frequent nut consumption and risk of coronary heart disease in women: prospective cohort study. BMJ. 1998;317(7169):1341-1345.

Simonte SJ, Ma S, Mofidi S, Sicherer SH. Relevance of casual contact with peanut butter in children with peanut allergy. J Allergy Clin Immunol. 2003;112(1):180-182.

Hourihane JO, Bedwani SJ, Dean TP, Warner JO. Randomized, double-blind, crossover challenge study of allergenicity of peanut oils in subjects allergic to peanuts. BMJ. 1997;314(7087):1084-1088

Cornelis MC, El-Sohemy A, Kabagambe EK, Campos H. Coffee, CYP1A2 genotype, and risk of myocardial infarction. JAMA. 2006;295(10):1135-1141.

Yang A, Palmer AA, de Wit H. Genetics of caffeine consumption and responses to caffeine. Psychopharmacology (Berl). 2010;211(3):245-257.

Womack CJ, Saunders MJ, Bechtel MK, Bolton DJ, Martin ES, Luden ND. The influence of a CYP1A2 polymorphism on the ergogenic effects of caffeine. J Int Soc Sports Nutr. 2012;9(1):7.

Winston AP. Neuropsychiatric effects of caffeine. Adv Psychiatr Treat. 2005;11(6):432-439.

Willoughby DS, Wilborn CD, Taylor L, Bressel J, Campbell WW. Performance and muscle function response to caffeine ingestion after 4 weeks of supplementation with 5 g/d creatine monohydrate. J Strength Cond Res. 2007;21(3):657-663.

Rogers PJ, Hohoff C, Heatherley SV, Mullings EL, Maxfield PJ, Evershed RP, Deckert J, Nutt DJ. Association of the anxiogenic and alerting effects of caffeine with adenosine A2a receptor gene polymorphisms. Neuropsychopharmacology. 2010;35(9):1973-1983.

Roehrs T, Roth T. Caffeine: sleep and daytime sleepiness. Sleep Med Rev. 2008;12(2):153-162.

References

Benton D, Greenfield K, Morgan M. The development of attitudes to chocolate questionnaire. Pers Individ Dif. 1998;24(4):513-520.

Goldstein ER, Ziegenfuss T, Kalman D, Kreider R, Campbell B, Wilborn C, Taylor L, Willoughby D, Stout J, Graves BS, Wildman R, Ivy JL, Spano M, Smith AE, Antonio J. International society of sports nutrition position stand: caffeine and performance. J Int Soc Sports Nutr. 2010;7(1):5.

Mort JR, Kruse HR. Timing of blood pressure measurement related to caffeine consumption. Ann Pharmacother. 2008;42(1):105-110.

Kanny G, Moneret-Vautrin DA, Parisot L, Daul CB. Food intolerance to wine. Allergy. 2001;56(3):211-212.

Vally H, Thompson PJ. Role of sulfite additives in wine induced asthma: single dose and cumulative dose studies. Thorax. 2001;56(10):763-769.

Clarke R, Bakker J. Wine Flavour Chemistry. 2nd ed. Wiley-Blackwell; 2011.

González de Llano D, Pascual-Teresa S, Martín-López MP, Ramírez-Tortosa MC, Barón-López FJ, Rivas-Gonzalo JC. Anti-inflammatory effects of a cocoa polyphenolic extract in rats. Food Chem Toxicol. 2010;48(10):2773-2780.

Jin D, Cao M, Wang W, Lin S, Chen Y, Zhu Z. Alcohol and its metabolic effects on liver: lipid and non-lipid metabolic pathways. Biomed Pharmacother. 2020;129:110388.

Vanderpump MP, Tunbridge WM, French JM, Appleton D, Bates D, Clark F, Grimley Evans J, Hasan DM, Rodgers H, Tunbridge F, Young ET. The incidence of thyroid disorders in the community: a twenty-year follow-up of the Whickham Survey. Clin Endocrinol (Oxf). 1995;43(1):55-68.

Haseeb S, Alexander B, Baranchuk A. Wine and cardiovascular health: A comprehensive review. Circulation. 2017;136(15):1434-1448.

Ginter E, Simko V. Moderate alcohol consumption and cardiovascular risk. Acta Medica (Hradec Kralove). 2013;56(1):7-12.

Cannon JG. Inflammatory Cytokines in Non-Pathological States. News Physiol Sci. 2000; 15:298-303.

Wantke F, Götz M, Jarisch R. Histamine-free diet: treatment of choice for histamine-induced food intolerance and supporting treatment for chronic headaches. Clin Exp Allergy. 1993;23(12):982-985.

DiNicolantonio JJ, O'Keefe JH. Dark chocolate: consumption for pleasure or therapy? Postgrad Med. 2017;129(6):637-638.

Holt RR, Lazarus SA, Sullards MC, Zhu QY, Schramm DD, Hammerstone JF, Fraga CG, Schmitz HH, Keen CL. Procyanidin dimer B2 [epicatechin-(4beta-8)-epicatechin] in human plasma after the consumption of a flavanol-rich cocoa. Am J Clin Nutr. 2002;76(4):798-804.

Russo GL, Tedesco I, Russo M, Cervellera C, Van Buren T, Schrijen F, van de Put F, Wiseman S, Hoffmann D, Koehler PE. Cellular antioxidant activity of flavonoid-enriched fractions from cocoa (Theobroma cacao L.): comparison with green tea (Camellia sinensis). J Agric Food Chem. 2004;52(4):433-438.

Stevenson DE, Hurst RD. Polyphenolic phytochemicals--just antioxidants or much more? Cell Mol Life Sci. 2007;64(22):2900-2916.

Bémeur C, Desjardins P, Butterworth RF. Neurobiology of alcohol-induced neurodegeneration. Alcohol Res Health. 2010;33(1-2):127-134.

Finley JW, Dewettinck K. Health aspects of chocolate. Crit Rev Food Sci Nutr. 2008;48(5):827-834.

West CE, Hammarström ML, Hernell O. Probiotics in primary prevention of allergic disease--follow-up at 8-9 years of age. Allergy. 2013;68(8):1015-1020.

Ros E. Health benefits of nut consumption. Nutrients. 2010;2(7):652-682.

Brennan L, Steffen L, Steinberger J, Daniels SR, Dolan LM, Mayer-Davis EJ, Prineas R, Jacobs DR Jr, Sinaiko AR. Relation of sweetened beverage intake to lipid and glucose abnormalities in children. J Pediatr. 2010;157(6):967-971.

References

Pasman WJ, Heimerikx J, Rubingh CM, van den Berg R, O'Shea M, Gambelli L, Te Riet L, Wopereis S, Hendriks HF. The effect of black tea on risk factors for cardiovascular disease: A randomized controlled trial. Arch Intern Med. 2010;170(7):699-705.

Gibson PR, Shepherd SJ. Personal view: food for thought—western lifestyle and susceptibility to Crohn's disease. The FODMAP hypothesis. Aliment Pharmacol Ther. 2005;21(12):1399-1409.

Staudacher HM, Lomer MC, Anderson JL, Barrett JS, Muir JG, Irving PM. Fermentable carbohydrate restriction reduces luminal bifidobacteria and gastrointestinal symptoms in patients with irritable bowel syndrome. J Nutr. 2012;142(8):1510-1518.

Barrett JS, Gibson PR. Clinical ramifications of malabsorption of fructose and other short-chain carbohydrates. Pract Gastroenterol. 2007; 31:51-65.

Ong DK, Mitchell SB, Barrett JS, Shepherd SJ, Irving PM, Biesiekierski JR, Gibson PR. Manipulation of dietary short-chain carbohydrates alters the pattern of gas production and genesis of symptoms in irritable bowel syndrome. J Gastroenterol Hepatol. 2010;25(8):1366-1373.

Halmos EP, Power VA, Shepherd SJ, Gibson PR, Muir JG. A diet low in FODMAPs reduces symptoms of irritable bowel syndrome. Gastroenterology. 2014;146(1):67-75.

Lehrer SB, Ayuso R, Reese G. Seafood allergy and allergens: a review. Mar Biotechnol (NY). 2003;5(4):339-348.

Turner PJ, Kemp AS, Campbell DE. Allergic reactions to food: what to do next. Aust Prescr. 2011;34(2):49-53.

Bernstein IL, Li JT, Bernstein DI, Hamilton R, Spector SL, Tan R, Sicherer SH, Golden DB. Allergy diagnostic testing: an updated practice parameter. Ann Allergy Asthma Immunol. 2008;100(3 Suppl 3)

.Daul CB, Morgan JE, Lehrer SB. Hypersensitivity reactions to crustacea and mollusks. Clin Rev Allergy. 1990;8(1):27-48.

Kelso JM. A tale of two controversies: diagnosing and managing "shellfish allergy" and the myth of "iodine allergy." Allergy Asthma Proc. 2009;30(5):466-468.

Matias BF, Vieira TF, Luz PB, Albuquerque TT, Borges LF, Cardoso MF, Grillo ZC. Glycoalkaloids in Solanaceae species. The good, the bad, and the bitter. Food Chem Toxicol. 2021; 152:112143.

Griffiths DW, Bain H, Dale MF. Solanine accumulation in potato tubers subjected to continuous illumination and cool temperatures. J Sci Food Agric. 1994;64(4):529-533.

Stamp LK, Chapman PT, Taylor WJ, Highton J. Tomato consumption is a trigger for some patients with gout. Rheumatology (Oxford). 2015;54(12):2275-2280.

Bharath LP, Jayawardena MT, Tyrrell DJ, Shivanna M, Goolcharan T, Venkatraman V, Sun Z, Unnikrishnan A, Whitehead N, Garvey SM, Maihle NJ, Qin Z, Roberts CK, De La Rosa A, Richardson RS, Zhang C, Amin RH, Jones DP, Gandhi H, Grote K, Ruderman NB, Griendling KK, Harja E, Go YM, O'Connor PM, Samsel PA, Sowers JR. Potatoes, tomatoes, and eggplants--oh my! An overview of glycoalkaloid toxins in nightshades and their potential health effects. Adv Nutr. 2019;10(4):604-616.

Luo W, Kooyers NJ, Pascali V, Bouniol AN, Munsch SH, Bouinot D, Calvino G. Capsaicin and its effects on health. Crit Rev Food Sci Nutr. 2021;61(5):735-760.

Part IV. Identifying Food Sensitivities

Benton D, Young HA. Reducing calorie intake may not help you lose body weight. Perspect Psychol Sci. 2017;12(5):703-714.

Matias SL, Greenberg SR, O'Leary MJ, Jones PR, Holt EM, Laing S, Weaver CM. Comparison of a short food frequency questionnaire with 4-day diet records in young women. J Acad Nutr Diet. 2020;120(1):117-124.

References

Gastrointestinal Symptoms, Food Sensitivities, and Hypersensitivity Disorders: A Practical Approach to the Gastrointestinal Workup. Am J Gastroenterol. 2019;114(6):936-946.

Vandenplas Y, Abkari A, Bellaiche M, Benninga M, Chouraqui JP, Çokura F, Harb T, Hegar B, Lifschitz C, Ludwig T, Morais MB, Özalp M, Polyviou I, Ribeiro H, Salvatore S, Shamir R, Singhal A, Shaoul R, Szajewska H, Vandenberghe N, Van Winckel M, Vieira M, Wabitsch M, Weghuber D. Prevalence and Health Outcomes of Functional Gastrointestinal Symptoms in Toddlers: A Pooled Analysis of Six European Countries. Pediatr Gastroenterol Hepatol Nutr. 2021;24(1):10-21.

Skypala IJ, Williams M, Reeves L, Meyer R, Venter C. Sensitivity-related illness: Nutritional assessment and dietary management. J Hum Nutr Diet. 2015;28(5):475-486.

Duncan H, Hill L, Evans P, Venter C. Dietary management of food allergy and intolerance in adults and children. Br J Community Nurs. 2015;20(12):606-611.

Gibson PR, Shepherd SJ. Evidence-based dietary management of functional gastrointestinal symptoms: The FODMAP approach. J Gastroenterol Hepatol. 2010;25(2):252-258.

Lee AR, Ng DL, Zivin J, Green PH. Economic burden of a gluten-free diet. J Hum Nutr Diet. 2007;20(5):423-430.

Ludvigsson JF, Leffler DA, Bai JC, Biagi F, Fasano A, Green PH, Hadjivassiliou M, Kaukinen K, Kelly CP, Leonard JN, Lundin KE, Murray JA, Sanders DS, Walker MM, Zingone F, Ciacci C. The Oslo definitions for coeliac disease and related terms. Gut. 2013;62(1):43-52.

Genuis SJ, Lobo RA. Gluten sensitivity presenting as a neuropsychiatric disorder. Gastroenterol Res Pract. 2014; 2014:293206.

Fasano A, Sapone A, Zevallos V, Schuppan D. Nonceliac gluten sensitivity. Gastroenterology. 2015;148(6):1195-1204.

Berin MC, Sampson HA. Food allergy: An enigmatic epidemic. Trends Immunol. 2013;34(8):390-397.

Kang JY, Lichtenstein DR, Steinberg WM, Schimmel EM. Non-celiac gluten sensitivity. World J Gastroenterol. 2021;27(7):639-653.

Fasano A, Catassi C. Clinical practice. Celiac disease. N Engl J Med. 2012;367(25):2419-2426.

Part V. Clear Skin Diet and Lifestyle Recommendations

Lunn J, Buttriss JL. Carbohydrates and dietary fibre. Nutr Bull. 2007;32(1):21-64.

Slavin JL. Dietary fiber and body weight. Nutrition. 2005;21(3):411-418.

Gibson RS, Bailey KB, Gibbs M, Ferguson EL. A review of phytate, iron, zinc, and calcium concentrations in plant-based complementary foods used in low-income countries and implications for bioavailability. Food Nutr Bull. 2010;31(2_suppl2)

Heseker H. Carbohydrate intake and prevention of nutrition-related diseases. Nutr Metab Cardiovasc Dis. 2001;11(4):205-221.

U.S. Department of Health and Human Services, U.S. Department of Agriculture. *Dietary Guidelines for Americans, 2020-2025*. 9th ed. December 2020.

Millward DJ, Garnett T. Plenary lecture 3: Food and the planet: Nutritional dilemmas of greenhouse gas emission reductions through reduced intakes of meat and dairy foods. Proc Nutr Soc. 2010;69(1):103-118.

Hoffman JR, Falvo MJ. Protein – Which is best? J Sports Sci Med. 2004;3(3):118-130.

Di Pasquale MG. The essentials of essential fatty acids. J Diet Suppl. 2009;6(2):143-161.

Mozaffarian D, Micha R, Wallace S. Effects on coronary heart disease of increasing polyunsaturated fat in place of saturated fat: A systematic review and meta-analysis of randomized controlled trials. PLoS Med. 2010;7(3)

References

World Health Organization (WHO). Diet, nutrition and the prevention of chronic diseases: Report of a joint WHO/FAO expert consultation. WHO Tech Rep Ser. 2003; 916:1-160.

Steinmetz KA, Potter JD. Vegetables, fruit, and cancer prevention: A review. J Am Diet Assoc. 1996;96(10):1027-1039.

Hoffman R. The Mediterranean diet: A health-promoting diet for all seasons? Nutrients. 2019;11(9):2089.

Guo Z, Xia J, Zou S, Fang Q, Zhang Y, Hou W, Zhang X. Associations between vitamin A, retinoid intake and risk of skin cancer: a meta-analysis. Int J Cancer. 2021;148(5):1007-1017.

Farris PK. Topical vitamin C: a useful agent for treating photoaging and other dermatologic conditions. Dermatol Surg. 2005;31(7 Pt 2):814-818.

Thiele JJ, Ekanayake-Mudiyanselage S. Vitamin E in human skin: Organ-specific physiology and considerations for its use in dermatology. Mol Aspects Med. 2007;28(5-6):646-667.

Umar M, Sastry KS, Al Ali F, Al-Khulaifi M, Wang E, Chouchane AI. Vitamin D and the pathophysiology of inflammatory skin diseases. Skin Pharmacol Physiol. 2018;31(2):74-86.

Zhang S, Shu XO, Li H, Yang G, Cai H, Gao YT, Zheng W. Vitamin K intake and the risk of cancer in the Shanghai Women's Health Study. Am J Epidemiol. 2010;171(7):800-805.

Suh H, Oh B, Kang DJ, Kim S, Kwon HJ, Park KY. The effects of biotin supplementation on skin hydration and other clinical outcomes in patients with atopic dermatitis: a randomized, double-blind, placebo-controlled trial. Ann Dermatol. 2020;32(1):43-49.

Ogawa Y, Kinoshita M, Shimada S, Kawamura T. Zinc and skin disorders. Nutrients. 2018;10(2):199.

Rayman MP. Selenium and human health. Lancet. 2012;379(9822):1256-1268.

Proksch E, Kaatz M, Kaczmarek M, Laquaz P, Segger D, Zague V. Oral supplementation of specific bioavailable collagen peptides improves nail growth and reduces symptoms of brittle nails. J Cosmet Dermatol. 2017;16(4):520-526.

Imai CM, Gunnarsdottir I, Thorisdottir B, Halldorsson TI, Palsson GI, Dagsson MH, Berven E, Jonsdottir I. Iron status and physical performance in a national cohort of adolescents: association between hemoglobin levels and cardiorespiratory fitness. PLoS One. 2018;13(2)

.Sanders ME, Benson A, Lebeer S, Merenstein DJ, Klaenhammer TR. Shared mechanisms among probiotic taxa: Implications for general probiotic claims. Curr Opin Biotechnol. 2018; 49:207-216.

Mikuls TR, Farrar JT, Bilker WB, Fernandes S, Saag KG. Suboptimal physician adherence to quality indicators for gout management. Pharmacoepidemiol Drug Saf. 2005;14(8):563-570.

Cohen PA. Probiotic use in clinical practice: what are the risks? Am Fam Physician. 2008;78(9):1073-1074.

Saghafi L, Rezaie M, Vahdat M, Sadeghi K, Eshraghian A, Razmpour F, Shekari M. Clinical applications of L-glutamine supplementation in the prevention and treatment of inflammatory bowel disease. Clin Nutr. 2021;40(2):586-593.

Moskowitz RW. Role of collagen hydrolysate in bone and joint disease. Semin Arthritis Rheum. 2000;30(2):87-99.

Richard C, Lewis ED, Goruk S, Field CJ, Jacques H, Ma DWL, McMurchy C, Muanza B, Baracos VE, Dinsmore MJ, Zello GA, Alenezi F, Widyaratna K, Curtis PJ, Field CJ. Marine- versus plant-derived omega-3 fatty acids differentially affect muscle inflammation and recovery following strenuous exercise. Clin Nutr. 2020;39(12):3536-3543.

Deshpande S, Nagendra HR, Raghuram N, Padmalatha V, Rao MV. A randomized control trial of the effect of yoga on gunas (personality) and self-esteem in normal healthy volunteers. Int J Yoga. 2009;2(1):13-21.

Khoury B, Sharma M, Rush SE, Fournier C. Mindfulness-based stress reduction for healthy individuals: A meta-analysis. J Psychosom Res. 2015;78(6):519-528.

Hirshkowitz M, Whiton K, Albert SM, Alessi C, Bruni O, DonCarlos L, Hazen N, Herman J, Adams Hillard PJ, Katz ES, Kheirandish-Gozal L, Neubauer DN, O'Donnell AE, Ohayon M, Peever J, Rawding R, Sachdeva RC, Setters B, Vitiello MV, Ware JC, and The National Sleep Foundation. National Sleep Foundation's sleep time duration recommendations: Methodology and results summary. Sleep Health. 2015;1(1):40-43.

American Psychological Association. Stress in America: Paying with our health. Stress in America Survey; 2015.

Tindel NL, Northrup RS, & Shaffer RA. Physical activity and exercise: Benefits of physical activity. Pediatr Rev. 2014;35(4):161-170.

Williams S, Kennedy G, Lanier C, Nieman DC. The impact of physical activity on human health: A focus on inflammation. Biochem Soc Trans. 2019;47(4):1105-1115.

Umberson D, Montez JK. Social relationships and health: A flashpoint for health policy. J Health Soc Behav. 2010;51(Suppl)

Seppala E, Simon-Thomas E, Brown SL, Worline MC, Cameron CD, Doty JR. The Oxford Handbook of Compassion Science. New York: Oxford University Press; 2017.

Brown KW, Ryan RM. The benefits of being present: Mindfulness and its role in psychological well-being. J Pers Soc Psychol. 2003;84(4):822-848.

Conclusion

Sharma M, Madaan V, Petty FD. Exercise for mental health. Prim Care Companion J Clin Psychiatry. 2006;8(2):106.

Dahlgren G, Whitehead M. Policies and Strategies to Promote Social Equity in Health. Stockholm, Sweden: Institute for Futures Studies; 1991.

Feldman R. The adaptive human parental brain: Implications for children's social development. Trends Neurosci. 2015;38(6):387-399.

Wright KP Jr, Drake AL, Frey DJ, Fleshner M, Desouza CA, Gronfier C, Kilgore L, Salameh W, Czeisler CA. Influence of sleep deprivation and circadian misalignment on cortisol, inflammatory markers, and cytokine balance. Brain Behav Immun. 2015; 47:24-34.

Calder PC. Omega-3 fatty acids and inflammatory processes: From molecules to man. Biochem Soc Trans. 2017;45(5):1105-1115.

Holick MF. The role of vitamin D for bone health and fracture prevention. Curr Osteoporos Rep. 2006;4(3):96-102.

Kelly GS. Quercetin. Monograph. Altern Med Rev. 2011;16(2):172-194.

Leung DY, Bieber T. Atopic dermatitis. Lancet. 2003;361(9352):151-160.

National Institute of Allergy and Infectious Diseases (NIAID). Guidelines for the Diagnosis and Management of Food Allergy in the United States. 2010.

Turnbaugh PJ, Ley RE, Hamady M, Fraser-Liggett CM, Knight R, Gordon JI. The human microbiome project. Nature. 2007;449(7164):804-810.

Images Credits

Leaky Gut and Dermatitis Herpetiformis images were purchased from Bigstockphoto.com.

All graphics, including cover design, were created by the author under supervision of Rima Petrosyan

ABOUT THE AUTHOR

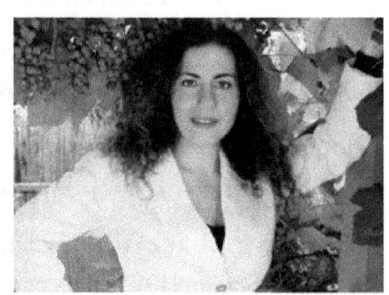

Dr. Azizian is a board-certified general surgeon and a certified functional medicine physician through the Institute of Functional Medicine. She is also a certified Root Cause Dermatology practitioner.

She founded Mindful Medical Care PC, a skin cancer clinic based in Falmouth, Massachusetts, and Mindful Medical Functional Clinic, an in-person and online clinic treating a broad spectrum of functional medicine conditions, including food sensitivities, functional dermatology, gut health, and more (www.mindfulmedicalfunctionalclinic.com).

With a passion for education, Dr. Azizian frequently speaks at conferences and events, covering a wide range of medical topics, from skin cancer to leaky gut. Her educational YouTube channel, **_Dr. Maria Azizian MD_**, is dedicated to skin conditions and functional medicine.

Her commitment to educating others stems from a deep belief that empowering patients with knowledge enables them to make well-informed decisions about their health care.

Dr. Azizian lives in Massachusetts with her husband and their three children.

The Clear Skin Diet: Unlocking the Secret Link Between Food Sensitivities and Skin Health is her second book.

www.ingramcontent.com/pod-product-compliance
Lightning Source LLC
Chambersburg PA
CBHW070612030426
42337CB00020B/3762